You're N

WASHINGTON'S HEALTH GUIDE FOR CAR ACCIDENT VICTIMS

Dr. David M. Warwick
Doctor of Chiropractic

Copyright © 2015 Dr. David M. Warwick

CreateSpace Publishing, Inc.

All rights reserved.

No part of this book may be reproduced in any form or by any electronic or mechanical means including information storage and retrieval systems, without permission in writing from the author. The only exception is by a reviewer, who may quote short excerpts in a review.

Printed in the United States of America
First Printing: October 2015

WASHINGTON'S HEALTH GUIDE FOR CAR ACCIDENT VICTIMS

For More Information Visit:

www.DrDavidWarwick.com

Facebook: Warwick Chiropractic PLLC
Google: Warwick Chiropractic
Instagram: drdavidwarwick
Yelp: Warwick Chiropractic

Table of Contents

INTRODUCTION 11

WHIPLASH AND BALANCE 26

THE MANY "FACES" OF WHIPLASH 28

WHIPLASH WHIPLASH: BODY, MIND AND SPIRIT – WHAT IS THE CONNECTION? 31

WHIPLASH AND LITTLE PROBLEMS 34

WHIPLASH – THE CAUSE OF PAIN 36

WHIPLASH WHIPLASH – CELL PHONES & OTHER DRIVING DISTRACTIONS! 39

WHIPLASH AND YOUR SENSE of POSITION & BALANCE 42

CHIROPRACTIC - "ONLY PROVEN EFFECTIVE TREATMENT" for CHRONIC WHIPLASH 44

WHIPLASH – THE IMPORTANCE OF SEATBELTS! .. 46

CAR ACCIDENT INSURANCE; ARE YOU COVERED? 50

WHIPLASH – CAN THIS AFFECT MY MEMORY? 52

THE WHIPLASH SYNDROME: CERVICAL TRACTION 55

NECK PAIN TREATMENT: RESULTS OF THE BONE AND JOINT DECADE 2000-2010 TASK FORCE ON NECK PAIN AND ITS ASSOCIATED DISORDERS 58

WHIPLASH – WHAT CAN I DO TO HELP? 60

WHIPLASH: WHERE'S THE PAIN COMING FROM?..63

AFTER MY CAR ACCIDENT, WHY DO I HURT SO MUCH? 65

WHIPLASH & CHIROPRACTIC TREATMENT.............68

CAN WHIPLASH HURT YOUR SHOULDER? 71

WHIPLASH –IMPORTANT POINTS TO KNOW!...........73

HOW TO IMPROVE YOUR ODDS OF CRASH SURVIVAL 76

WHIPLASH MAJOR STUDY QUESTIONS THE USE OF MUSCLE RELAXANTS, PAIN MEDICATIONS, AND NSAIDS IN WHIPLASH INJURIES 79

WHIPLASH – WHAT IS IT? 82

WHIPLASH: WHAT ARE THE ODDS OF A PERMANENT INJURY?..85

WHIPLASH AND TREATMENT DELAY: DOES IT MATTER?..88

WHIPLASH MINIMIZING YOUR RISK FOR WHIPLASH 90

WHAT CAUSES WHIPLASH? 92

WHIPLASH-ARE YOU COVERED? 95

WHIPLASH WHIPLASH ASSOCIATED DISORDERS .97

WHIPLASH – WHAT IS THE BEST TYPE OF TREATMENT? 100

INTERESTING FACTS ABOUT WHIPLASH 103

WHIPLASH AND YOUR LIGAMENTS 106

WHIPLASH! DO I NEED AN ATTORNEY? 108

THE WHIPLASH SYNDROME 111

MILD TRAUMATIC BRAIN INJURY – WHAT'S THAT? 114

THE WHIPLASH SYNDROME: RINGING IN THE EARS 117

WHAT REALLY CAUSES WHIPLASH? 120

MORE WHIPLASH FACTS 123

WHIPLASH: CAN IT BE PREVENTED? 126

WHIPLASH - BIOMECHANICS AND COSTS 129

WHIPLASH - WHO WILL RECOVER? 132

WHIPLASH - WHICH TREATMENT METHOD IS BEST? 135

CAR ACCIDENTS AND MILD TRAUMATIC BRAIN INJURY 138

WHIPLASH AND VISION - WHAT'S THE CONNECTION? 141

EVEN MORE WHIPLASH FACTS..........................144

WHIPLASH AFTER AUTO ACCIDENTS WHIPLASH DOWN THE ROAD..147

WHIPLASH INJURY AND CERVICOGENIC HEADACHE..149

WHIPLASH DIAGNOSIS...153

HOW CAN I GET HURT IN A LOW-SPEED CRASH?..156

WHIPLASH AND SIDE COLLISIONS......................158

WHIPLASH AND PTSD...161

WHAT MOST PEOPLE DON'T KNOW ABOUT CAR ACCIDENT INJURIES..164

WHAT CAN I DO TO HELP MYSELF?......................166

THE WHIPLASH SYNDROME: POSTURE AND EXERCISE 171

DON'T TAKE OUR WORD FOR IT, HERE'S WHAT OUR PATIENTS HAVE TO SAY ABOUT FEELING BETTER FAST™ AFTER AN ACCIDENT…...............................174

Introduction

If you have been recently injured in a car accident, you are probably confused and worried about what to do next. I bet you are asking yourself questions like the following:

"Will my car be repaired?"
"Will my medical bills be paid?"
"Will I ever get better?"
"Will I be paid for the time I'm missing from work?"
"What do I do if the other person doesn't have car insurance?"
"What will the insurance company offer me for my injuries?"

If you or someone you care about has any of these concerns, please keep reading this special Car Accident Victim's Guide. My name is David M. Warwick, D.C, and I've been helping injured people get fast relief from auto accident injuries in Lacey / Olympia for almost 20 years.

Whiplash injury is a **"very real"** problem that costs communities billions in health care and disability dollars.

Studies have recently shown that about 10-20% of the population suffers from neck pain, and car accidents/traumas are a big cause of this type of pain.

But you've probably wondered how something as minor as a fender-bender to your bumper could be such a pain in neck.....

Maybe your doctor told you "give it a couple of weeks"..."you'll be fine."

But you're not fine.

Your neck hurts when you work at the computer, when the dog pulls too hard on the leash... maybe sleep has become more difficult with a lot of tossing and turning, or you've become dizzy...or always tired when you used to be full of energy and pep.

Maybe you've noticed how your neck moves differently since the accident. Looking over the shoulder perhaps isn't as easy as before.

Does all of this sound familiar?

It's quite surprising when you look at whiplash research and its global impact-the entire body is affected. You probably didn't think that headaches or fatigue were part of the whiplash bargain, but they are.

Your Bumper Doesn't Tell the Whole Story...

You can't look at a dent in the bumper and conclude that the neck wasn't injured.

For instance, they're called 5 mph bumpers for a reason-designed to not be damaged in very low speed collisions.

This is good for the bumper, but not necessarily for your neck!

What researchers have discovered is that when collisions are of enough force, this causes the vehicle to crumple and absorb energy. Low speed collisions will often not cause the crumple zones to be engaged.

If you have a rigid fixed bumper (seen on many older cars and trucks), that does not crumple-this can make the whiplash injury even more severe.

For the above reasons, you might be even more injured in an accident below 20 mph than one above that speed.

There are of course limits to this effect. Collisions at very high speeds (above 40 mph) will often cause the occupants to suffer severe injuries, even though the crumple zones are absorbing some of the energy.

You may have heard someone profess skepticism for your whiplash injury. Maybe they thought you were gaming the system or out to make a fast buck. Where does this perception come from?

Probably the insurance companies, who may have a profit-motive for denying the realty of whiplash injuries.

Some physicians are simply ignorant about whiplash trauma, perform cursory spinal examinations, or offer treatments that have little or no scientific evidence to back them up.

But is there really such a thing as "Whiplash?"

The science says, "YES!"

Whiplash-a soft tissue injury to the neck-is also called neck sprain or neck strain.

It is characterized by a collection of symptoms that occur following damage to the neck, usually because of sudden extension and flexion.

The disorder commonly occurs as the result of an automobile accident and may include injury to the joints of the spine, disks, and ligaments, cervical muscles, and nerve roots.

Symptoms such as neck pain may be present right after the injury or may be delayed for several days... especially days 3, 4 and 5 after the accident.

In addition to neck pain, other symptoms may include:

- Neck Stiffness
- Injuries to the Muscles and Ligaments (Myofascial Injuries)
- Headaches
- Dizziness
- Abnormal Sensations Such As Burning or Prickling (Paresthesia)
- Shoulder Pain
- Back Pain

In addition, you may be experiencing cognitive, somatic, or psychological conditions such as:

- Memory Loss
- Poor Concentration
- Nervousness/Irritability
- Sleep Disturbances
- Fatigue or Depression.

But Why Can Whiplash Be So Devastating?

Your head and neck is simply not designed to be accelerated three times the acceleration of gravity....or come in contact with an air bag deployed at 190 mph.

When these injuries occur, muscles and ligaments of the neck cannot resist the force, which then tears tissues apart. This then sets the stage for degeneration/osteoarthritis years later.

The basic principal in a rear-end whiplash, is anything that makes your vehicle not accelerate as fast when hit, is going to make the injury less damaging to your neck.

If your car is small, it will accelerate much more quickly than a larger vehicle.

If you're hit on a low friction surface such as rain-drenched pavement, or ice, the car will accelerate very quickly...and some of the worse injuries occur when your vehicle is slightly rolling when hit, because it's easier to get a vehicle moving that is not stopped.

Women are more injured by whiplash, because they generally have less neck musculature development. The ratio of their head size to their neck size is much greater than in a man. There's a very good reason why professional football players have those massive necks.

The Four Dangerous Whiplash Myths:

Myth #1: Car Damage = Occupant Injury

It might seem intuitive that if a car is smashed, the neck will be badly injured, and conversely if it's a simple fender bender, then the neck was spared. Some low speed collisions can be even more damaging than high-speed accidents, within certain limits. The kinds of things that may be more important are if your head is turned, or the size of the vehicle that is hitting you.

Before the accident, was the vehicle was rolling or stopped, how was the headrest positioned? Other factors include getting hit from behind vs. a head-on impact.

Research shows that people are not as badly injured from frontal impacts. It could be the airbag, anticipating the collision and tightening up, or the chin hitting the chest. All other factors being equal it's worse to get hit at the side and behind, than at the front.

Airbags have done a lot to save lives from frontal collisions. Unfortunately, side and rear impacts are less protected by an airbag. Seatbelts also save lives by keeping the occupants inside of the vehicle. Although they save lives, they tend to actually accentuate whiplash injuries in low speed collisions where the torso is more restrained relative to the head and neck.

Even car seats can be a factor in how badly you're injured. Cars with soft thick seats will cause the head to whip more than occupants in a thin firm seat. If the headrest was placed too low, it will act as a fulcrum and make the neck injury much worse. That's why your headrest should always be positioned at the very highest level, and just touching the back of the head.

Myth #2: No Pain = No Injury

I don't feel pain so I'm ok. Most people who get in an accident will feel flustered and shook up. In low speed collisions, it is rarer to have pain right after accident. Usually symptoms develop over days, and it is not uncommon for the pain to come on two weeks post trauma. Conversely if you feel immediate pain, then substantial tearing and damage has occurred.

Another thing to consider is that the spine can be injured and yet may not cause much neck pain. However, these patients usually have tender spines to the touch, even if there are no outward symptoms. Less than 20% of the nerves that come through bundles between your vertebrae carry pain signals.

That means it's important to examine for more than just pain, such as neurological and muscle function. A doctor needs to carefully palpate the tissues of the neck, check range of motion, and examine the flexibility of individual spinal joints. With this type of comprehensive exam you will be able to know if you've been injured.

Myth #3: Kids Don't Get Whiplash

Kids aren't injured in whiplash. Maybe you thought little Johnny wasn't injured in the car seat, or since kids tumble around when they play, they couldn't possibly be injured. This couldn't be further from the truth.

Infants and young children have much undeveloped spines with much less muscle strength. This makes their ability to resist the forces lessened. You have to also consider the size of the head compared to the size of the neck. This difference is greatest in young children.

When infants are injured they *can* show behavioral changes such as irritability and disrupted sleep patterns or nursing difficulties.

Myth #4: X-rays Always Show Whiplash Injury

If you've had a severe whiplash, you may have taken a trip to the emergency room where an x-ray was taken. If you're like many patients, the x-ray was read as normal. The problem is the x-ray you received, probably taken with you in one position, does not show injuries to the soft tissues such as ligaments and muscles, unless massive injury has occurred. Only if motion x-rays are obtained, can you see how the joints are moving in the neck. Since the injury is a sprain of ligaments, and x-rays show only bones-they do not give the complete picture.

Unfortunately for some whiplash victims, Neck trauma will lead to arthritis of the spine.

Don't be too alarmed, but concern is helpful. People hear the word arthritis and think of rheumatoid arthritis and crippling joints. What I'm talking about is osteoarthritis, or degenerative joint disease.

Osteoarthritis is one of most common diseases afflicting humans, more common in people over age 55 than any other health condition.

Billions of dollars are spent each year on drug treatments that really do nothing to prevent degeneration of the joint. In fact, some scientists suggest that injuries do not heal properly when patients take NSAIDs such as ibuprofen. This is in addition to the known rare side effects such as stomach bleeding, liver, and kidney problems.

Arthritis occurs in spinal joints that have damage to the ligaments and disks. As degeneration progresses, the mobility of vertebrae are altered. The stretched out ligaments will allow excessive motion and after injury, scar tissue develops. Over months and years, the scar tissue contracts and the disk size decreases. This will make the mobility of the neck abnormally low (more stiffness). This scar tissue is also not as elastic as tissue that has not been injured. Persons, who have pre-existing degeneration and arthritis at the time of impact, will suffer whiplash more frequently and with more severity when it does occur. Since older adults are most likely to have this type of degeneration arthritis, they are put more at risk in whiplash accidents.

One of the mainstays of medical treatment of whiplash is to immobilize the neck with a collar. Except in rare cases, it is something that I never use in practice.

While good in theory, it just weakens the muscles and fails to preserve movement, which the neck needs to heal properly.

I am glad to see that many medical physicians are using them less and less, and promoting more active rehabilitation. Neck collars/braces are needed for fractures or dislocations, but strains/sprains are generally made worse with this treatment. In fact, recent studies show that 90% of patients, who are fitted with a collar, end up with arthritis!

I have spent years studying the mechanics of neck problems, and effective treatments, and I've successfully cared for many patients over the years, getting their quality of life back and reducing pain. But I'm still surprised by how many still take the medical approach-hot packs, collars and pain pills.

Treatments ideally should be mechanical, not chemical, and not just cover up or mask the pain.

I'm not saying that I have all the answers. But I do think there is a general lack of appreciation for the seriousness of these types of neck injuries, and that people are often convinced by insurance companies and others, that no injury occurred.

This can sometimes result in no examination, no professional treatment, or the patient self-medicates with various over-the-counter drugs or maybe you were required to see a "gatekeeper," that didn't appreciate the complexities of whiplash injuries and never referred you to the appropriate doctor.

Not seeking proper treatment when indicated can lead to more problems down the road. The most crucial point I want you to get from this book, is that...

You Are In The Right Place!

Also, one of the most common questions our office gets after someone is involved in an accident and sustains injuries is:

Do I Really Need An Attorney?

Choosing the right attorney may be critical for your case. Insurance company adjusters are trained to handle claims as quickly and cheaply as possible. You may need a professional negotiator on your side to help walk through the process and ensure you get the claim you deserve.

I have seen patients receive offers from their insurance company to settle for $1500 when a good personal injury attorney might have gotten them 10 times that! All you are looking for is a fair settlement to help provide for any future medical bills, lost time from work, as well as pain and suffering, and an attorney trained in personal injury can make sure you get just that!

How Do I Choose An Attorney?

It can be very difficult to know what attorney is right for you. First, you want to select an attorney who specializes in personal injury cases. If you wouldn't go to a dermatologist for heart surgery, then why would you go to a tax attorney to help with your personal injury claim? It sounds silly, but many people assume that just because their next door neighbor or friend from church went to law school that they can help them negotiate a personal injury claim.

There are lots of good attorneys in the Lacey / Olympia WA area that have helped my patients with their auto accident cases. My office can provide you with names of good, honest attorneys who will make sure you get the compensation you deserve!

I also want you to know that it is very important for you to follow your Chiropractors recommendations over the first 6-8 weeks after the accident, in order to ensure that you have the absolute best chance of avoiding arthritis or degenerative disc disease.

Over the past almost 20 years I have treated hundreds of patients with whiplash injuries, and I believe the systematic approach we use in my office to be very effective at helping patients Feel Better Faster.

Don't take my word for it.....I have included a sample of my many satisfied patients that have written testimonials. I have also included a collection of the most relevant articles I have published in my popular "In Good Hands" newsletter over the last few years.

It's easy to make your first appointment with me. All you have to do is call my office today at **(360) 951-4504** and schedule an evaluation to see if we can help you. We'll do everything possible to get you in the same day...even if we have to stay late or work through lunch! You're too young to suffer with terrible auto accident injuries. Let's handle them today. Ok, here's what to do right now…

Call (360) 951-4504 Today!

My staff and I would love to work with you. All you have to do is call my office right now and we will schedule a time that's convenient for you! I have the friendliest staff you will ever meet and we are all specially trained in handling the often-confusing paperwork and forms that need to be filled out.

We look forward to helping you Feel Better Faster.

David M. Warwick, D.C.

This book has been carefully prepared to educate those who have suffered-whiplash types of injuries of the neck and spine. The information presented is for general health education only. Individual health concerns should be addressed with a knowledgeable and licensed health care provider.

Whiplash and Balance

As whiplash injuries are studied more and more, the many health problems that can develop as a result of them are becoming more apparent. Neck sprains are not simple problems like a sprained ankle because the neck is involved in a lot of important duties, not just movement. One such function of the neck is to keep you upright and in balance. Balance is complex and involves coordination between sensations in your inner ear, your eye movements and neurological signaling from your neck, spine and legs. The neck nerves are especially important in this regard. The brain receives inputs from the ears, the eyes, and neck, and determines from these three areas where you are in space, where've you been, and where you are going. If any of these areas is affected, then balance is disturbed.

You may stumble around more, not really have a sense of where your feet are; you may trip more and in severe cases, you may develop vertigo (a spinning sensation). These symptoms can have a devastating effect on your quality of life, even resulting in nausea.

A recent study from Europe (funded by an insurance company) (Coll Antropol 2007;31:823) looked at how we sense position of the head following whiplash. The researchers compared whiplash-injured patients to normal healthy people in their ability to sense the position of their head; whether they were rotated or tilted in some way. The results were alarming. Patients with cervical spine injury showed significant impairment of proprioception (sense of position)

Chiropractic care involves trying to normalize joint function of the neck. Adjustments are designed to restore normal mobility and improve the posture of the neck so that it is more balanced. Some patients will need specific exercises, even balance therapy, to help improve their sense of position and keep them from feeling dizzy.

So if you've wondered about feeling unsteady, or are not really sure on your feet, this could be a consequence of a whiplash injury. Because both the brain and neck can be injured in whiplash, the symptoms can be quite substantial. Just letting it go and hoping it will go away can create an even longer lasting problem. And bed rest or simply not moving the neck are not good treatment options after an auto accident either, because your neck needs to move to properly heal. Some neck collars can even create more of a problem leading to muscle weakness. They are right for some patients, but not for everyone.

The Many "Faces" of Whiplash

Motor vehicle collisions (MVC) usually result in injuries to the neck and upper back. However, there are often other complaints that can occur immediately or after a delayed time frame. The mechanism of injury or, "how did the accident happen?" is very important to discuss in detail. For example, a **low speed crash** such as 5-10 mph may not result in much damage to the car. However when this occurs, the contents inside the car are jostled and thrown about more than if there had been car damage. This is because the impact was too slow to dent or crush the metal and the energy of the crash was not absorbed but rather, transferred to the contents inside the car – that is, the passengers.

Another cause might be a roll-over accident. If a person is suspended upside down in the vehicle, injury can occur from the seat belt, from falling from the seat upon releasing the seat belt, cuts or scrapes from broken glass, and so on. Many people involved in MVC's are initially in "shock" and may **not realize they are hurt until hours or three, four or even five days later**. Upon rising the next morning, a significant increase in pain intensity often prompts the person to seek emergency room care where medications are usually prescribed and a "wait and watch" recommendation is given. Within the initial several days to a week, gradual **increases of pain and other symptoms** such as headaches, dizziness, "foggy thinking," and loss of appetite due to the high pain intensity can occur, and the person may then visit a chiropractic clinic, as the "waiting and watching" approach just doesn't make sense any longer.

The initial examination findings often reveal **significant muscle spasms** and pinching of the nerves in the upper part of the neck, resulting in headaches.

Patients may have difficulty describing their complaints including problems communicating with others such as, "I just can't find the words I want to use." This lack of mental clarity is often caused by a concussion and can last weeks to months. Some patients do well and may feel 50-75% better after 3-6 weeks of chiropractic treatment with respect to neck pain and headache intensity and frequency but of course, this varies from patient to patient. During this time, exercises are usually given to help stretch the tight muscles and strengthen the weak muscles in the neck and upper back region. **Temporary work restrictions may be required**, especially if the patient had not been able to work prior to seeking chiropractic treatment. A quick return to work is usually very important.

Hence, **a "wait and watch" approach usually does not work very well**. In addition, the use of medications may prohibit being able to drive a car or adequately function at work. Certain medications can also affect a person's ability to responsibly manage their children. The primary goal of the chiropractic physician is to achieve a reduction in symptoms and return the patient to a productive, functional lifestyle as quickly as possible.

Whiplash: Body, Mind and Spirit – What is the Connection?

The term "whiplash" refers to an injury to the neck muscles, the muscle attachments (tendons), ligaments, and sometimes the disks that lie between the vertebral bodies of the spine. In a rear-end collision, the cause of whiplash occurs from a sudden, rapid acceleration of the body and neck as the car is pushed forwards. In these first 50-75 milliseconds following impact, the head remains in the same place while the body is propelled forward. This is followed by a "crack-the-whip" movement of the head and neck when the muscles in the front of the neck stretch like rubber bands and suddenly spring the head forwards, all occurring in less than 300 msec. The force on the head and neck is further intensified if the seat back is too springy, or angled back too far. Also, if the headrest is too low, the head may ride over the top and more injury can result.

The treatment of whiplash varies from "watchful waiting" to a multidisciplinary team approach that includes neurology, physical therapy, chiropractic, psychology, and possibly surgery (rare). In a recent article published in the American Journal of

Physical Medicine and Rehabilitation (2009, March Vol. 88, No. 3, pp 231-8), the relationship between clinical, psychological and functional health status factors was investigated in a group of patients with chronic whiplash-associated disorder (WAD). A total of 86 patients with chronic WAD participated in the study and outcomes were tracked using questionnaires that measure pain, disability and psychological issues including depression, anxiety and catastrophizing. Physical examination factors included measuring the cervical range of motion. An analysis of the degree of neck disability and the relative contribution of physical vs. psychological factors revealed catastrophizing and depression played greater roles than did cervical range of motion. This suggests psychological factors play an important role in the outcome of whiplash.

The importance of this is that more than just the physical factors like range of motion should be focused on when treating chronic whiplash patients. Answering the patient's questions, explaining the mechanism of injury and how that relates to their specific condition, and addressing depression, anxiety, coping, and other psychological issues is very important. Discussing treatment goals with patients is also very important. For example, making light of the injury by stating something like, "...you'll be fine after the treatments," may harm the patient as anything short of "fine" may be interpreted as failed treatment by the patient. It is also important not to paint too dismal of a picture as that can have negative psychological effects as well, as this may suggest that they will never improve. Explaining the difference between "hurt" and "harm" is of great value to the chronic whiplash patient as they are often told, "if it hurts, don't do it." This sends an unfortunate message to the patient that any activity where an increase in pain occurs is "bad" when in fact, that activity may help the patient get better in the long run. This can make or break an acceptable outcome as many may feel like they shouldn't do anything and this can lead to unemployment, boredom, and the many psychological issues previously described. The best advice is to remain active and try to ignore discomfort by staying within "reasonable activity boundaries." Reasonable activity tolerance is learned as time passes and trying different activities for different lengths of time.

Whiplash and Little Problems

I find myself educating patients daily about the function and posture of the neck. I really enjoy letting my patients know about something so important to their health. I just wish more people knew this information from an early age. If they did, they would pay more attention when their neck stiffens or when they bump their head. These little things don't seem to be of much consequence when they happen but little things do add up over time.

Even a simple car accident may not seem like much if no blood was involved or the vehicle only had a small dent in the bumper. But these little problems do end up having consequences, and the x-ray usually shows these effects. When I review a patient's x-rays, there are sometimes changes that had to occur years earlier. It is often the beginning stages of arthritis with disk degeneration. If you recently injured your neck in a car accident, this pre-existing degeneration may have made your less able to withstand the forces of the collision. But it also indicates you had a little problem years earlier. Perhaps the body gave you a signal at the time, a stiff neck or even minor pain but the pain gradually went away and you thought the problem did as well.

Unfortunately, the body may not heal completely on its own and over time if the posture of the neck is ignored or the mobility isn't preserved, the small joints of the spine can wear out, sort of like tires wearing unevenly on a car that is out of alignment.

It surprises me sometimes how well we take care of our cars, changing the oil regularly, having it aligned, but when it comes to the spine; even a collision with a wall is thought to be of little consequence.

If your neck is letting you know something isn't quite right, maybe stiffness, pain or headaches, it's important to get it checked out after an auto accident. Working on your posture at an early age and keeping your mobility even and smooth are best taken care of early on, not after arthritis has set in.

Whiplash – The Cause of Pain

Many patients ask the question: *"...why do I hurt so much now, and hardly hurt at all right after the accident?"* Another common question is: *"...why neck pain after a minor car collision can last so long?"*

A study that investigated chronic pain and dysfunction in whiplash cases reported a soft tissue origin for injuries associated with low-speed collisions. This means the pain comes from the muscles, ligaments, joint capsules, the disk, but not from a pinched nerve that would send pain down the arm and/or create hand numbness or grip weakness.

The study also reported the point at which the neck buckles would only take one fifth to one-fourth of the weight of the person's head (approximately 2.5 to 3 pounds) if one were to remove all of the supporting muscles, ligaments, and joint capsules. With the muscles and soft tissues intact, there is a very complex buckling pattern that occurs in the neck during most rear-end collisions where the lower half of the neck bends opposite to that of the upper half creating an S-shaped curve (when looking at the neck from the side).

When this occurs, the vertebrae in the lower half of the cervical spine extend backwards while the upper half flex forwards, stretching the ligaments beyond the maximum elastic point and tissue tearing occurs. When ligaments stretch or strain, microscopic tearing starts at only 3-5% of tissue strain and when the strain reaches 7-8%, the ligament begins to lose its load carrying capacity and more significant tearing occurs. Unfortunately, none of this can be seen on a standard x-ray and usually goes undiagnosed.

Many variables exist that make assessing the amount of tissue damage difficult to predict or understand. One of these variables is the strength and amount of elasticity of a ligament prior to tearing. Also, the age, gender, and phenotype – that is, skinny, normal, or over weight – makes a difference.

Generally, due to a reduced muscle mass in a female compared to most males, women are at greater risk of injury. The position of the person in the car, whether a seatbelt was used or not, if the head was turned before impact, if the collision was anticipated prior to impact, the speed at which one person compared to another can voluntarily contract a muscle are all additional factors affecting the degree of injury and corresponding pain. Another factor is the size of the spinal canal (the place where the spinal cord runs from the brain to the low back) as some people are born with narrow canals, making them more susceptible to injury.

Other neurological variables include the degree of the excitability of the nervous system as the more excitable, the lower the pain threshold and pain is perceived more quickly. The type of pain from the deep tissues (ligaments, joint capsules, etc.) is different than pain arising from superficial tissues as the former lasts longer and doesn't follow known neurological pathways into an arm. Also, over time, if pain becomes chronic (pain lasting >3 months), a significantly lower pain threshold is found in these cases vs. normal control subjects.

Whiplash – Cell Phones & Other Driving Distractions!

Whiplash is caused by a sudden movement of the head, usually caused by a motor vehicle collision (MVC) but it can also occur in sports and from slip and fall injuries. The combination of the weight of the head (approximately 15 pounds) and the length and strength of the neck predisposes the neck to be injured when a sudden force is applied. This is also caused by the fact the neck muscles cannot tighten quickly enough to prevent injury in these types of injuries. People with slender necks (i.e., women > men) are more prone to injury.

The purpose of this article is to discuss some VERY effective ways to reduce the likelihood of being in a MVC of which the obvious include don't drink and drive, don't use your cell phone and drive, and doesn't "text" on your phone while driving. Instead, use a hands-free phone or better yet, pull over to talk as you can't concentrate or fumble around dialing/texting, and still pay proper attention to what you're supposed to be doing – that is, driving!

According to a study conducted by the University of Utah, the distraction resulting from talking on a cell phone when driving is more significant than being intoxicated (0.08% blood-alcohol). Driving inattentively is estimated to be a factor in 20-50% of all police-reported MVC's of which 8-13% are caused by driver distractions (cell phones is estimated to be 1.5-5% of that). One study reported both hands-free and hand-held cell phones were similar, reducing the driver response time to about a 40th percentile compared to a "normal driver."

It's believed the "cognitive workload" or, the "thinking" part during conversation causes the primary distraction, not the use of the hands. When compared to talking with a passenger, the University of South Carolina reported planning to speak put far more demands on the brain than listening. Talking to other passengers or on a cell phone are not the only or, the most common of the driving distractions.

The two most common causes of distraction-related accidents are "rubbernecking" (looking at outside objects/events) and adjusting the car radio/CD player. Cell phone use was reportedly 8th on that list. The use of a cell phone to text is limited because it is relatively new. However, a preliminary report from the University of Utah found a 6-fold increase in distraction related accidents when texting. The obvious concerns include the eyes off the road and in some cases, the hands off the wheel required for texting/email. Of interest, about 50% of drivers between 16 and 24 years of age compared to 22% of 35-44 year olds have admitted to texting while driving. Some recent highly publicized MCV's caused by texting drivers include a May 2009 Boston trolley car driver and, the 2008 Chatsworth train collision that killed 25 people.

A July of 2009 Virginia Tech report of video footage of 200 long haul truck drivers who drove over 3 million combined miles, reported 81% of safety critical events involved driving distractions. They found texting had the greatest relative safety risk at 23 times more likely with their eyes being off the road for 4.6 out of a 6 second during a safety critical event. Another significant cause of driver distraction is drowsiness, which increased the driver's risk of a crash or near-crash by 4 times, reaching for a moving object increased the risk by 9 times, looking outside/rubbernecking = 3.7 times, reading = 3 times, applying makeup = 3 times, dialing a cell phone = 3 times and talking or listening on a hand-held devise = 1.3 times. Eating while driving is also a risk.

Whiplash and Your Sense of Position & Balance

Although whiplash injuries are quite common, research is only beginning to describe the diverse symptoms that can develop when the neck has been traumatized. Even minor whiplash such as occurs from sports, can have a significant impact on the delicate structures of the neck.

Position sense or balance is how we keep upright and move through space. When it is disturbed we may feel unsettled, dizzy or even get nauseous. Many studies have shown that when the spine is injured, the person's balance can be affected. How is this so? Balance is maintained by a complex interaction between your inner ear, your eyes, and the nerves in your neck (Sports Med 2008;38:101,Armstrong. et al.). When the neck is injured you may use your eyes more to make up any position sense or balance deficits. There are limits to this strategy and as a result dizziness is a big problem in society. About 1/3 of older persons suffer from dizziness, and whiplash or other neck traumas can be a significant factor.

A good test to see if your balance is impaired is as follows: Can you stand on one leg for fifteen seconds? Is it equally easy to do this on the other leg or is one side easier to maintain your balance. Can you stand on one leg with your eyes closed? Obviously you should try this very carefully. You may want to do this with a friend nearby so you do not fall. Do you immediately lean and have to put your other foot down? If you cannot stay upright it may be sign that position sense has been affected by a spinal problem.

Chiropractic care can improve the posture and mobility of the neck. This may have an impact on balance because joint dysfunction in the neck can send altered nerve signals to brain centers that coordinate position with your eyes and ears. Although there is limited research in this area, most doctors and therapists recognize the importance of introducing movements when a balance problem is coming from a neck injury. It's important to introduce limited movements early following a trauma as long as additional pain is not being provoked.

Chiropractic – "Only Proven Effective Treatment" for Chronic Whiplash

You might have wondered, "Who should I go to for treatment of my whiplash problem?" You have many choices available in healthcare ranging from drug related approaches such as narcotic medications to natural forms of treatment such as chiropractic, exercise, and meditation with many others in between. Trying to figure out which approach or perhaps combined approaches would best serve the needs of the presenting patient is truly challenging. To help answer this question, one study reported the superiority of chiropractic management for patients with chronic whiplash, as well as which type of chronic whiplash patients responded best to the care. The research paper begins with the comment from a leading orthopedic medical journal stating, "Conventional treatment of patients with whiplash symptoms is disappointing." In the study, there were 93 patients divided into three groups consisting of:

1) Group 1: Patients with a "coat-hanger" pain distribution (neck and upper shoulders) and loss of neck range of motion (ROM), but no neurological deficits;

2) Group 2: Patients with neurological problems (arm/hand numbness and/or weakness) plus neck pain and ROM loss; and,

3) Group 3: Patients that reported severe neck pain but had normal neck ROM and no neurological losses.

The average time from injury to first treatment was 12 months and an average of 19 treatments over a 4 month time frame was utilized. The patients were graded on a 4-point scale that described their symptoms before and after treatment.

- Grade A patients were pain free;
- Grade B patients reported their pain as a "nuisance;"
- Grade C patients had partial activity limitations due to pain; and
- Grade D patients were disabled.

Here are the results:

<u>Group 1</u>: 72% reported improvement as follows: 24% were asymptomatic, 24% improved by 2 grades, 24% by 1 grade, and 28% reported no improvement.

<u>Group 2</u>: 94% reported improvement as follows: 38% were asymptomatic, 43% improved by 2 grades, 13% by 1 grade, and 6% had no improvement.

<u>Group 3</u>: 27% reported improvement as follows: 0% was asymptomatic, 9% improved by 2 grades, 18% by 1 grade, 64% showed no improvement, and 9% got worse.

This study is very important as it illustrates how effective chiropractic care is for patients that have sustained a motor vehicle crash with a resulting whiplash injury.

Whiplash – The Importance of Seatbelts!

Whiplash is a very common problem afflicting millions of people each year. In fact, there are more than 6 million car accidents each year in the United States alone. Death associated with car accidents occurs every 12 minutes and each year, motor vehicle collisions (MVC) kill 40,000 people. For people aged between 2 and 34 years old, MVCs are the leading cause of death.

Another sobering statistic is somebody is injured in a car crash every 14 seconds and about 2 million people receive permanent injuries in car crashes each year. Over a five-year period, over 25% of ALL drivers were involved in a motor vehicle collision. The cost of car accidents averages $1000 for each American per year resulting in a $164.2 billion total cost each year in the United States.

Approximately 250,000 children are injured and car crashes, meaning approximately 700 kids are injured daily. Car crashes are the leading cause of acquired disability. Hopefully, these rather startling statistics have gotten your attention. Last month, we discussed various effective ways of reducing the likelihood of even being in a motor vehicle collision (MVC). As an appropriate follow-up, this discussion will cover seatbelts and their role in injury prevention and life-saving capabilities.

In general, the available evidence available is clear – seatbelts save lives! Regarding backseat passengers, wearing a seatbelt is 44% more effective at preventing death than riding unrestrained. Similarly, for those positioned in the rear of a van or sport utility vehicle, the use of rear seatbelts is 73% better at preventing a fatal outcome during a car crash.

In more than one half of all fatal car accidents, the victims are not properly restrained. The National Highway Traffic Safety Administration (NHTSA) in 2008 reported the use of seatbelts increased 1% over 2007 with 83% of drivers wearing their seatbelts. The use of seatbelts increased to 90% on highways versus 80% on surface streets (in town).

In states where rear seatbelts are required, 85% of adult backseat passengers complied versus states not mandating rear seat seatbelt use where only 66% of the passengers complied. The NHTSA has launched a campaign, "Click It or Ticket" and has provided a guide to seatbelt safety promoting the proper use of the seatbelt and have provided the following safety seatbelts tips:

- Make sure your seat belt fits snugly. Seat belts worn too loosely can cause broken ribs or injuries to your abdomen.

- Place the lap belt low on your hipbones and below your belly. Never put the lap belt across your belly.
- Place the shoulder belt across the center of the chest between the breasts.
- Never slip the upper part of the belt off your shoulder. Seat belts that are worn too high can cause broken ribs or injuries to your belly.
- The most effective safety protection available today for passenger vehicle occupants is lap/shoulder seat belts combined with air bags.

There is a common myth that seatbelts cause injuries at low speeds and therefore, it is better to not wear the seatbelt when simply traveling in town. There is overwhelming evidence in almost all circumstances, seatbelts save lives, even at low speed collisions. Because the forces that occur in low-speed crashes are transferred to the contents due to the lack of crushing metal and less vehicle damage, the occupants of a car struck at a low speed can be thrown about significantly… striking the windshield, side window and other contents inside the car.

Car Accident Insurance; Are You Covered?

Most states require drivers to carry various types of insurance to protect themselves as well as others who may be involved in an unfortunate accident. Drivers, and the banks that may carry the car's loan, generally think of the vehicle first when deciding on appropriate coverage. While it's difficult to think about, you need to also consider whiplash injuries to you and your passengers, and potentially other drivers and passengers, should you be determined to be at fault. Some drivers also carry medical insurance (med pay), which can be accessed for care in the event of an auto accident.

Some items to consider are that vehicle repairs can be quite costly, as can health care. If you are the cause of a multi vehicle accident, minimal amounts of insurance may not cover the costs of repairs for expensive new vehicles. In terms of health care, an ambulance ride with minimal interventions could cost $1000-$1,500 dollars. If you spend a few hours or a day in an emergency room, this could run into the thousands, especially if advanced imaging such as MRI or CT scans are needed. This is just the beginning of your evaluation in a severe accident. Then, there are the costs of whiplash treatment over perhaps months, disability from being able to work and other costs. If a few passengers are involved, the costs can soar.

It's important to discuss these issues with your insurance agent. Is your med pay adequate? Sometimes med pay premiums are a cost-effective way to get some additional piece of mind. A $1,000.00 med pay allowance will not last long in today's health care environment. Chiropractic care, while very cost effective compared to medicine or surgery, can still run into the thousands if severe whiplash injuries have resulted from the auto accident in Las Vegas. You may also need to consider uninsured and underinsured coverage should another driver be at fault and not adequately insured.

If you've been involved in an auto accident, it's important to get evaluated right after an injury to get you Feeling Better Faster.

Whiplash – Can This Affect My Memory?

"Doctor, is it normal for people after a whiplash injury to notice problems with memory. I can't seem to remember things I just recently did since my car accident?"

This is a common complaint occurring as a result of a whiplash injury, but it's not commonly known, leaving those who are suffering wondering, *"...what's wrong with me?"* Whiplash is an injury that classically occurs as a result of a car crash at any speed, even at low speed! This is because at low speed, there is little to no damage to the car, and the forces from the crash are not absorbed by the crushing metal. As a result, those forces are transferred to the contents inside the car – that is, the passengers. This sometimes results in a significantly greater injury compared to crashes that occur at twice the speed because the latter results in crushing metal.

The actual injury that occurs in whiplash is caused by the sudden, rapid movement of the head resulting in varying degrees of injury to the neck, as well as to the contents inside the skull – that is, the brain. The brain literally "bangs" into the inside walls of the skull when the head is rapidly accelerated during a car crash. The resulting injury is a concussion. What's interesting is that most patients injured in a car crash often don't mention a concussion nor is it usually asked about at the doctor's office as other, more obvious injuries are dwelt with. The condition is usually referred to by one of two names: post-concussive syndrome or mild traumatic brain injury (MTBI).

"Doctor, when I'm reading a book or magazine, sometimes I have to re-read the passage several times before it sinks in. It's as though I lose my concentration and I can't focus on what I just read. The other day, I was talking to a group of co-workers and I lost my place in the middle of the discussion and had to ask, '...now where was I?' I notice this is happening a lot since the car accident."

This can be very embarrassing, frustrating, and scary for patients suffering with MTBI. Other symptoms associated with this include difficulty in focusing (blurred vision), headaches, having difficulty in pronouncing certain words ("tongue twisted"), having difficulty in understanding what was said, difficulty remembering numbers or groups of numbers like phone numbers, addresses, birthdates, and so on.

These symptoms can range from mild to severe and can be very disruptive, making work and everyday tasks challenging.

How long does it last? MTBI can completely clear up in 2 to 6 months without problems or, it can hang on for 2 years or longer, and may even become a permanent residual from the car crash. In one study, continued problems after a 2 year time frame were reported in close to 20% of those injured 2 years earlier. This study suggests that about 1 out of 5 may continue to suffer with MTBI and the associated brain-related problems for at least 2 years following a car crash. However, another study reported the long term "higher cognitive function" (such as the ability to communicate through written or spoken language) is usually not affected by whiplash injuries. However, they preface that with by reporting that a more commonly injured group with more mild brain problems was found.

As chiropractors, we are trained to do a thorough history, orthopedic and neurological examination, and ask specific questions about mild traumatic brain injury. It is important to discuss this information with those suffering from whiplash injuries as frequently, MTBI patients think something is "...seriously wrong" and harbor unnecessary anxiety.

The Whiplash Syndrome: Cervical Traction

Whiplash injuries include damage to the soft tissues of the neck such as muscles, tendons, ligaments, and myofascial tissues. The degree of injury is typically graded on a 1-3 scale from least to most tissue damaged, respectively. A grade 1 sprain (ligament injury) or strain (muscle or muscle tendon injury) includes minimal tissue disruption or tearing while grade 3 sprains and strains include significant tissue tearing and subsequently longer healing times with greater chance of long-term residual problems.

More severe whiplash injuries can result in fracture but those types of injuries are not indicated for traction forms of therapy until after the fracture heals and stability is restored to the neck. So, the question is what role does cervical traction play in the management of neck pain associated with whiplash?

In whiplash injuries, when it feels good to the patient to have someone pull on their neck, that person is a candidate for cervical traction. The amount of weight or traction force and length of time are based on patient comfort and are highly variable. Therefore, it is important to start with a low enough weight so injury to the patient from the traction therapy is avoided. Typically, 5#/15 minutes is a safe starting point, gradually increasing the weight to a maximum tolerated level.

Many insurance companies, based on the published literature regarding cervical traction, regard it as a "medically necessary" form of treatment and hence, a covered service. There are many different cervical traction devices available for home use of which the over-the-door traction unit is typically the least expensive and in some cases mandated prior to insurance allowance for a more expensive pneumatic cervical traction device.

Unless there are reasons that over-the-door traction is not tolerated such as jaw pain (due to the chin strap pressure), this approach is commonly utilized. This device includes a water bag that is calibrated for water weight and can be done multiple times a day, depending on each case.

There is also a collar-type of traction unit which allows the patient to move around rather than sit in one place. However, the amount of weight is better regulated with the water bag/sitting type. There are laying down types of neck traction which can also be regulated accurately for weight. These tend to be more expensive and insurance companies may require use of the less expensive over the door type first, unless there is a medical reason that a chin strap is not tolerated.

Below are pictures of the different types of units available:

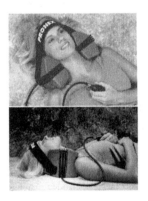
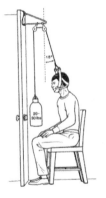
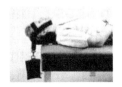
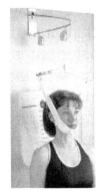

Neck Pain Treatment: Results of the Bone and Joint Decade 2000-2010 Task Force on Neck Pain and Its Associated Disorders

Whiplash and neck pain are complex injuries involving the delicate soft tissues and the nerves of your neck. Usually, motor vehicle accidents are responsible for these types of traumas. Even low-speed collisions can produce significant injury. People with these types of injuries may have central or back pain, arm pain, and even headaches or dizziness/vertigo. Some people with minor muscle strains will recover quickly but a large percentage will develop chronic problems leading to suffering that can last for months or even years.

Many different doctors, such as chiropractors and medical physicians, osteopaths and surgeons, provide treatment for whiplash pain with a wide variety of methods. It is important to sort out which treatments really work from those that are costly, useless, or even harmful.

In addition to whiplash treatments provided by doctors, there are many physical therapists, personal trainers, masseuses and any number of home remedies that people seek out in trying to get some relief for their severe pain. To a patient faced with all of these different options in can seem quite daunting to decide which approach to choose since all can seem reasonable. It would be nice if doctors could come to some agreement rather than forcing patients into the health care maze.

Fortunately researchers have recently brought some attention to this complicated field. The prestigious medical journal SPINE recently published the results of a best-evidence review of all treatments for neck pain (Hurwitz, et. al. Spine 2008;33:S123-52). The Bone and Joint Decade Task Force reviewed literature of non-invasive treatments (no surgery) from 1980 through 2006. A total of 139 papers were considered scientifically valid for review and covered treatments such as educational videos, mobilization (deep stretching movements), manual therapy (done by hand), low level laser therapy, exercises, and acupuncture. In addition to pain relief, the scientists also considered costs and safety. Their conclusion was that the best treatments for accident related whiplash injuries involving manual therapy and exercise are more effective than alternative strategies for patients with neck pain.

Whiplash – What Can I Do To Help?

Whiplash occurs when the neck is suddenly and forcefully jerked, and is typically associated with car crashes. The speed at which the neck is forced upon impact is faster than we can contract our muscles in attempt to stop the forceful movement. This results in muscle, tendon, and/or ligament over-stretching, even tearing. Symptoms include stiff and painful neck movements, weakness or, the head "feels heavy" making it challenging to "hold up" as well as headache, and sometimes dizziness, ear noises, TMJ or jaw pain, and "mental fog." What should be done if a whiplash injury occurs?

The amount or degree of damage to the soft tissues – that is, the muscles, tendons, ligaments, and disks of the neck -- will be the deciding factors as to how much rest vs. activity should be initially performed. If there are no fractures, dislocations or other injuries resulting in an unstable cervical spine (neck), studies have shown rest and a soft collar is actually harmful when compared to early return to activity and exercises. Chiropractic treatment, which essentially exercises the joints of the neck, has been shown to speed recovery when performed sooner rather than later after a whiplash injury. A handy way to classify the injury includes four categories: 1) Pain with no significant abnormal clinical findings; 2) Pain with mild clinical findings and range of motion loss; 3) Pain with neurological injury (resulting in radiating arm pain); and 4) Pain associated with fracture and/or dislocation. Those suffering with category 1 or 2 injuries should minimize rest, collar use, proceed with life's activities and not be afraid to do desired activities. More aggressive exercise and, utilizing chiropractic adjustments as soon as possible are very effective in the first two categories of injury. Category 4 (fractures and dislocations) injuries require the use of a rigid collar usually for 4-6 weeks as rest/protection is imperative. Category 3 demands careful monitoring by your chiropractor as neurological problems like arm pain and numbness, muscle strength weakness, must be watched during the healing process. The use of ice is helpful with all four categories of injury and exercise training is important and can be started sooner in the first two categories of injury.

What can you do if you sustain a whiplash injury? The first order of self-help is the use of ice. This is a much better choice over the use of heat as ice reduces swelling and pain while heat can increase swelling because it brings in more blood flow into an already swollen area. The heat may feel good during its use but most patients report the pain either returns shortly thereafter or feels worse. Ice and heat can be alternated but ice should be emphasized by using ice for 10 minutes, heat 5 minutes, and repeat the ice / heat / ice approach starting and ending with ice. One session usually equals 40 minutes (ice/heat/ice/heat/ice for 10+5+10+5+10, respectively, = 40 min.), and several sessions can be repeated each day. "Contrast therapy" of ice/heat/ice/heat/ice can be performed for as long as there is pain or, for several weeks or longer. The good news is that you will never hurt yourself by using ice but, you might make it hurt worse by using heat too soon so, when in doubt, use ice right after the injury! The next, very important, recommendation is to utilize exercises to stretch and strengthen the neck and upper back region. The "general rule" of exercise is slow repetitions staying within "reasonable" boundaries of pain. That is, a good, stretch type of pain is encouraged while avoiding sharp pain.

Whiplash: Where's the Pain Coming From?

Whiplash commonly occurs as a result of a motor vehicle collision when, typically, there is hyper-motion in one direction followed by motion in the opposite direction in a "crack the whip" like manner.

The direction of the strike typically dictates the direction of movement of the head so in a rear end collision, the strike is from behind, whipping the head forwards and then backwards. In a side-on collision, a side-to-side motion results. Pain can occur anywhere around the neck, upper back, arms, chest and/or head, depending on the tissues that are injured. Soft tissues including the muscles, their tendon insertions, ligaments that securely tie bone to bone, the shock absorbing disk in the front of the vertebral column, and/or the nerves that pass through the holes of the spine that innervate the arms and hands can be affected by these injuries.

There can be jaw pain, difficulty in swallowing, balance / dizziness problems, fatigue, as well as concussion or mild traumatic brain injury which can lead to poor concentration, sleep interference, and memory loss. Low back pain and/or trunk pain can occur from the seatbelt and/or airbag deployment.

The injuries associated with whiplash can lead to disruption of normal daily activity, depression and anxiety. There can be immediate symptoms or a delay in the onset and pain with its associated disability can last for days, weeks, months, or longer, depending on each case.

Last month, we discussed the grades 1, 2, and 3 or, mild, moderate, severe sprains (ligament injuries) and strains (muscle injuries). Previously, we discussed methods of prognosing the lasting effects of the injury in a reported classification system called "whiplash associated disorders" or WAD I, II, III. & IV. Here, the differentiating feature is pain with no objective exam findings (WAD I), the presence of objective loss of motion but negative neurological findings (WADII) or, the presence of measurable neurological dysfunction (WAD III). Studies have shown that the likelihood of prolonged injury increases with each WAD grade.

A side-to-side or front-to-back mechanism of injury can result in damage to the ligaments in the back of the spine called the supra- and inter- spinous ligaments, the disk and/or nerve root that exits the spine allowing the arm and hand to sense and be strong (when it's not pinched or damaged like in a WAD III) and/or, the bone which can compress when the force is hard enough (WAD IV). A concussion can occur when the brain bounces against the inside of the skull.

After My Car Accident, Why Do I Hurt So Much?

There are many different reasons why injuries sustained in car crashes result in chronic or long term pain. First, there are several types of tissues in the neck that can give rise to pain. The most intense pain comes from the tissues with the greatest density of nerve fibers, such as the joint capsules and the ligaments holding the bones of the neck together.

There are many ligaments in the neck that are vulnerable to being over-stretched and injured in a motor vehicle collision. The mechanism of a "whiplash" injury in a rear-end collision is unique. Upon impact, the vehicle rapidly accelerates forward while the head momentarily remains in its original position, resulting in an initial straightening of the neck followed by extension. At the extreme end-range of backward extension motion, the ligaments in the front of the neck are over stretched and can tear.

Within milliseconds, the head is then propelled forwards into flexion which can then injure the ligaments in the back of the neck placing a significant amount of force on the joint capsules and ligaments holding the bones in close proximity. Another reason the neck is injured is the speed at which the head and neck "whip" in the backwards and forwards directions after the impact. This occurs faster than what we can voluntarily contract our neck muscles to resist--within 600 milliseconds! Therefore, even if we brace ourselves in preparation for an impact, we can't avoid injury to the ligaments and joint capsules.

Damage to the ligaments is difficult to "prove" by conventional x-ray, which is why bending views or, flexion/extension x-ray methods are needed. When there is damage to the ligaments, the vertebra will shift forwards or backwards excessively compared to neighboring vertebra. This can be measured to determine the extent of ligament laxity or damage and can help explain why neck pain can be so intense and/or chronic.

Not all car accidents occur from behind. In fact, only about 1/3 occurs from this direction. One study investigating which direction created greater degrees of injury reported 57% of chronic pain patient group occurred from rear-end collisions. It also found that woman sustained more ligamentous injury compared to men and that frontal and rear end collisions resulting in significantly higher levels of ligament injury compared to side impacts

Another well published reason why neck pain can "hurt so much" after a car crash is that the sensory input from the injured area to the brain can be so extreme that it leaves an "imprint" in the sensory portion of the nervous system and it becomes hypersensitive or sensitized, resulting in a lower pain threshold or being more sensitive to pain. This is similar to the "phantom limb" phenomenon that often occurs after a leg is amputated where the brain still "feels" leg pain after the limb has been removed.

This has also been reported to be a reason for the significant constellation of symptoms often accompanying "whiplash" injuries. A partial list of associated symptoms with whiplash injuries includes neck pain, headache, TMJ / jaw pain, dizziness, coordination loss, memory loss, cognitive difficulty in formulating thought, communicating, losing your place during conversation, and more.

Chiropractors have a unique advantage over other health care

providers as manual therapies, including spinal manipulation, have been shown to yield higher levels of satisfaction and faster recovery rates compared to other forms of health care. We pride ourselves in performing thorough history and physical examinations, offering high quality evidence-based therapeutic approaches and teaching necessary home-based, self-management procedures.

Whiplash & Chiropractic Treatment

How many patients who sustain a whiplash injury actually improve and recover compared to those that don't? In one study, it was stated that 43% of patients will suffer long-term symptoms after a whiplash type of injury. More specifically, if a patient is still symptomatic after 3 months following the injury, "...then there is almost a 90% chance that they will remain so."

They go on to state that no conventional treatment has proven to be effective in helping these chronic cases. The purpose of their study was to determine the effectiveness of chiropractic treatment in a group of chronic whiplash patients. To do this, they studied 28 patients (20 women and 8 men, between ages 19-66, mean 39) over a 2-year time frame, injured in motor vehicle collisions.

Their symptom severity was graded on an A to D scale (A=minimal symptoms vs. D=disabling symptoms, with B= nuisance and C=Intrusive or partially disabling). Those in Groups C & D either had to significantly modify their work or, they lost their jobs and relied on continual use of medications.

The chiropractic treatment included spinal manipulation (adjustments), controlled resistance of muscles to improve stability and coordination, and the use of ice. Treatment from an emergency facility and/or their general practitioner and physical therapy had been previously utilized for on average 15.5 months, before entering this chiropractic-based study.

Initially, 27 of the 28 were classified into symptom groups C or D and symptoms included neck pain (82%), neck stiffness (36%), and other complaints of headache, shoulder, arm and back pain. Following treatment 26 of the 28 (93%) improved 16 by one symptom group and 10 by two symptom groups and this degree of improvement was assessed and agreed upon by both an orthopedic surgeon as well as by a chiropractor. Seventeen (61%) improved to a point of satisfaction where care was discontinued after the 1st assessment with 4 of the 17 considering return for treatment due to a return of symptoms. Litigation was still pending in 20 of the 28 cases at the time the study concluded.

This study is very important as over 90% of chronic whiplash cases improved from chiropractic management well beyond the point of improvement obtained through standard emergency, family practice and physical therapy. Other studies have pointed out that early intervention or treatment with chiropractic manipulation and management approaches generally results in a more favorable response compared to waiting for longer time periods. To be able to obtain this level of success after an average of 15.5 months is truly remarkable!

Chiropractic methods often utilized for patients with a "whiplash" injury include spinal manipulation (or adjustments), mobilization techniques (this includes stretching, figure 8 movements, manual traction), muscle release work (this includes trigger point therapy, myofascial release/friction massage, and others), and promoting self-help approaches (this includes exercise, home traction methods, computer station modifications and other job modifications as indicated, and others).

Can Whiplash Hurt Your Shoulder?

It's probably more common than you think. Whiplash injuries, especially serious ones, are notorious for causing pain and disability beyond the neck. Whiplash is considered a full body disorder and symptoms can range from pain to dizziness, headache and fatigue.

Depending on the type of collision and restraints, other body parts may be injured as well. One study (Abbassian A, Giddins GE. Sub acromial Impingement in patients with whiplash injury to the cervical spine. J Orthopedic Surgery 2008;3:25.) looked at shoulder complaints in individuals who had suffered a whiplash type of trauma. Out of 220 patients with whiplash, 26% had shoulder symptoms and 5% had what is known as an impingement syndrome.

Referred pain from the neck and nerve injury to the muscles that stabilize the shoulder can give rise to an impingement syndrome. Also, direct trauma from the pressure supplied by a seatbelt during a frontal impact can cause fracturing of cartilage and sprain of the surrounding ligaments. The pointy top of the shoulder is the acromium and some impingements (binding and compression) can affect the tendons of the rotator cuff or other soft tissues just under this bone. Sometimes a bursa (fluid filled sac) can swell during the night causing pain.

Because most patients with whiplash who have shoulder pain are thought to have referred pain from the neck, an impingement syndrome may be overlooked. This can delay treatment, resulting in prolonged disability, pain, and chronicity.

An MRI may be needed to fully diagnose the problem and confirm the lesion. Sometimes the labrum, cartilage surrounding the bone, can break away causing significant pain. There may be inflammation surrounding the different tendons as they are caught between the shoulder bone and the soft tissues. Most shoulder injuries can be conservatively treated and rarely require surgery.

Chiropractors are trained to differentiate between neck and shoulder problems and provide specific treatments to each area. Sometimes, an adjustment may be needed to align the shoulder joint or neck. In other cases the shoulder can be helped by specific exercises for the rotator cuff muscles. The important part of this issue is first getting the problem properly diagnosed. If you don't know what is causing the pain, it is nearly impossible to have a specific, effective solution.

Whiplash–Important Points to Know

What Is It? Whiplash is an injury to the soft tissues in the neck including ligaments, joint capsules, muscles and their tendons, and intervertebral disks. It can also involve the nervous system tissues in more severe cases, resulting in radiating arm pain.

How does it happen? During a car crash, most commonly a rear-end collision. The sudden jolt occurs so fast we cannot brace ourselves adequately and the head accelerates back and forth beyond the limits of the ligaments that hold our bones firmly together (often referred to as a "sprain"). Because of the significant range of motion of the neck, the weight of the head, and how is suspended on the neck, the neck is particularly vulnerable to this type of injury (more commonly worse in woman due to a more slender neck).

What are the symptoms? The primary symptom is neck or upper back pain that may develop immediately or be delayed days, weeks, and sometimes months. A partial list of possible symptoms (each injured person's symptoms are different) include: muscles spasms, loss of movement, headache, dizziness, concentration &/or memory loss, difficulty swallowing, chewing &/or hoarseness, burning or tingling, shoulder/arm/hand radiating pain, and more.

How is it diagnosed? Even when symptoms do not seem significant, a health care provider can diagnose the condition by taking a careful history and performing a physical exam. X-rays showing a change in the curvature or contour of the neck, &/or MRI or CT scan to better assess the disk and nerve roots when pain radiates down an arm may also be indicated. When persistent concentration/memory loss is present, a consult by a neuropsychologist is helpful.

How is it treated? In most cases, non-surgical methods are usually appropriate. If you go to a medical doctor, typical approaches include a wait & watch approach and/or medications such as anti-inflammatory drugs, pain killers, &/or muscle relaxants. MD's may refer the patient to physical therapy. When these methods fail, referral to a physiatrist may result in injection therapy (epidural steroid, facet injection, trigger point injections). Chiropractic care includes spinal manipulation, mobilization, soft tissue release techniques, exercise training, activity modification training, and physical therapy modality use (electrical stimulation, traction, ultrasound, TENS unit). Care may also include a mix of provider approaches, when appropriate.

How can it be prevented? The degree of severity of whiplash can be decreased or maybe avoided completely with the following: the use of seatbelts (especially in high speed collisions), placing the headrest close to the head (< 1 inch) and high enough to avoid "ramping" over it. Placing the seat back more vertical/upright can minimize ramping. Do not partake in distractive activities while driving – cell phone use, adjusting the radio, taking your eyes off the road (eye contact during conversation), dosing off, reading a book (this is more common than you think!), and others. Bracing yourself has not been shown to be very helpful – whiplash happens too quickly to voluntarily brace your neck muscles. For athletes, wear appropriate protective gear when engaging in sporting activities and use proper form / technique during the athletic activity.

Important to know! Chiropractors have a unique advantage over other health care providers as spinal manipulation and other manual therapies have been shown to yield the highest levels of satisfaction and faster recovery rates compared to other forms of health care.

How to Improve Your Odds of Crash Survival

You might ask, what does this headline have to do with chiropractic? It's often said case management or patient care is much more than just what we do to our patients (such as in chiropractic, applying a spinal adjustment). The patient education portion of our care plan can frequently make or break a successful outcome in a case. It is the goal of this Health Update to potentially save your life by empowering you with the knowledge needed when it's time to purchase your next car. This is about what specific automobile features contribute to crash survival – hence, saving lives!

Did you know the car you choose can improve the odds of crash survival by 400%? In the popular magazine Consumer Reports, they wrote, "Ultimately, safety is active and passive, balancing the ability to avoid an accident and to survive one." Typically, the first thing we do as consumers when we consider safety in a particular car is to look at the crash-test results. While this is important, we must first consider the size and weight so we compare crash-test results between cars in the same weight class since statistics show there are two times as many occupant deaths annually in small vs. large cars. Keeping size and weight in the foreground, when evaluating crash-test results, the front and rear end "crumple zone" of the car should be designed to absorb crash forces by buckling and bending in a serious collision. If you've ever watched race cars crash, you usually see car parts bend and break off as they bounce off the guard rail or other cars, sometimes to the point where all that is left is the cage surrounding the driver. Amazingly, the race car driver often climbs out of the cage and walks away, seemingly unharmed.

The next important car feature to consider is a car with a structurally superior passenger compartment. Look for a high quality "restraint system" made up of 3 components: seat belts, airbags, and head restraints. This work together to keep us safe and in place during a crash while the outside of the car crumples, absorbing the energy of the crash.

So where do you look to get this information? There are several resources available:

- The NHTSA (National Highway Traffic Safety Administration) tests front end impacts at 35 mph, and in 1997 added side impact tests at 38 mph. They also test for the rollover potential for SUVs and trucks and grade the results for each category from 1 to 5 stars representing the likelihood of suffering a life-threatening injury in a crash.
- Since 1995, the IIHS (Insurance Institute for Highway Safety) has used a method reviewed by Consumer Reports as being more realistic by crashing only half of the vehicle at similar speeds into fixed barriers, since most crashes are not direct, whole car strikes.
- Consumer Reports is a 3rd option. They integrate the data from both NHTSA and IIHS and gives us their "CR Safety Assessment," and run 40 new cars each year through numerous individual tests.

Other important "accident avoiding" features often overlooked include:

Tires - greatly impact braking and emergency handling so REPLACE them as needed;

Braking-check for the distance required to stop the car at different speeds- the shorter, the better;

Emergency Handling-data about accident avoidance and choosing a vehicle with electronic stability control (ESC), especially in SUVs is wise;

Acceleration-the quicker a car can get to highway speeds, the better;

Driver position and visibility-a good view of the surroundings, especially the "blind spots" is important.

Whiplash Major Study Questions the Use of Muscle Relaxants, Pain Medications, and NSAIDs in Whiplash Injuries

A scientific review published recently (Chochrane Database Syst Rev, July 2007) casts doubt on many common whiplash treatments. Despite billions spent on scientific research each year for the best treatments for whiplash injuries, it is surprising that many common treatments lack valid scientific evidence for safety and effectiveness. As studies accumulate in libraries, some groups take an interest in figuring out the data landscape and what it all means for doctors, and more importantly, the patients they serve.

Researchers from the Chochrane group did just that, and retrieved studies that took place over the past two decades. They specifically looked at medical treatments in whiplash and other mechanical neck disorders. It was all a bit of a disappointment because of surprisingly few studies, and when they were actually conducted, were of very limited quality-meaning it was hard to reach conclusions. An area of evidence that was especially weak, was studies of muscle relaxants (these relax muscles), analgesics (these block pain signals), and nonsteroidal anti-inflammatory drugs/NSAIDs (these reduce inflammation). The authors concluded that their benefits are not proven in solid scientific studies and that any potential benefits are "unclear."

Of course this report received little media attention, and we continue to see advertisements on TV and in print that tell patients to go for a pill to help their mechanical neck pain or whiplash pain. Rarely are viable options such as conservative chiropractic care discussed. Most patients who get whiplash injuries in

Lacey / Olympia follow the medical approach of drugs and sometimes even surgery.

Perhaps you may want to consider a mechanical approach for a mechanical problem such as whiplash after an auto accident. Or maybe you've had some doubts about consuming many medications over several months or even years. When consumed over long periods of time, NSAIDs in particular can lead to stomach bleeding and other complications such as liver and kidney problems. Although an ad on television may state that, "simple blood tests are needed to check for liver problems," liver problems such as liver failure are anything but simple.

And of course just simply blocking pain signals is unlikely to get at the cause of your pain, which is usually a sprain of the small joints of the spine.

Whiplash – What Is It?

Whiplash is a slang term for an injury to the neck that occurs as a result of a sudden jolt, classically occurring in a car accident though a slip and fall injury can sometimes result in a similar condition. In a classic rear-end collision, the car is struck from behind and accelerated forward at speed that even if the person knew the impending collision was about to take place, bracing the body prior to impact would not prevent injury.

In fact, muscles can only be voluntarily contracted at around 800-1000 msec. and in a rear end collision; the head is "whipped" within a 300-400 msec. time frame. Add to that, the muscles in the front of neck are initially stretched with the car is propelled forward leaving the head in a relatively extended backwards position.

Most of the headrests in cars are not properly positioned so the head often goes back much farther than the limits of our muscles, ligaments and joints may allow resulting in stretching and tearing of these tissues. When the tissues in the front of the neck are over stretched, the "rubber band" effect propels the head forward --

overstretching the muscles, ligaments, and joints in the back of the spine.

This "crack the whip" phenomenon occurs within 400-500 msec., far quicker than what we are capable of when voluntarily contracting our muscles. Here is a breakdown of what happens in a 5 mph rear-end collision:

0 msec.: At the moment of impact, the car seat just begins to move and the occupant has not yet been accelerated forward.

50 msec.: As the back of the car seat pushes the torso forward, the spine moves forward, resulting in a straightening of the thoracic and cervical spine. About 2-3 G's of force are exerted on the torso.

75 msec. This difference in motion between the neck and torso results in an S-shaped curve, where nearly all of the bending in the cervical spine takes place in the lower cervical spine. This rapid bending in just a few joints can result in ligament damage in the lower spine.

150 msec.: Here, the torso has pulled so far forward on the lower neck that the head is forced backwards often over the head restraint. Depending on the position of the headrest, the angle of the seat back, and "spring" effect of the seatback, the ligaments in the front portion of the spine are often injured during this phase of the collision. About 3-4 G's are exerted on the shoulders.

200 msec. Finally, the force of the car seat throws the head and torso forward. Here, 5 G's are exerted on the head and neck as it whips forwards. All of this is completed in less than 500 msec.

One of the reasons this occurs has to do with the ability of the car – particularly the back bumper to not deform so that the force of impact is transferred directly to the contents within the vehicle (i.e., the passengers). At higher speeds, the crushing metal absorbs some of the impact and the contents are actually less jostled and thrown about. This helps explain how a no damage rear end collision can result in greater injury than a higher speed collision.

Whiplash: What Are The Odds of a Permanent Injury?

I'm sure you've heard someone claim, "...you're not really injured – you're just going for a big settlement!" Or, "...that person isn't really hurt, they're just in it for the money!" Though there are cases that may fit this scenario, the majority of people who are injured in a motor vehicle collision would gladly forfeit any settlement to have their health and sometimes their life back. So, where in this process does the truth lie? Do most people "fake" their complaints or, are they really in pain? And, is there a way to determine who is more likely to suffer with problems long after their case is settled?

To answer this question, the Quebec Task Force (QTF), published two studies to investigate what types of whiplash injuries, which they term "whiplash associated disorders" (WAD), sustained in a rear end or side impact motor vehicle collision might end up with no residual injury vs. those more likely to become permanently disabled or impaired. The first of the two studies published in 1995 introduced 3 categories of injuries:

- Those with neck pain, stiffness or tenderness only - no clinical (exam) findings;
- Neck complaints and clinical findings including decreased ranges of neck motion;
- Neck complaints and loss of neurological function including numbness or weakness in arm strength and/or altered reflexes.

The QTF then set out to investigate whether this approach could indeed accurately predict those more vs. less likely to end up with significant disability with ongoing problems. They published these results in 2001 and found if they broke down the 2nd category into two groups, those with vs. without neck motion loss, those patients who fell into the 2nd group (with neck motion loss) and the 3rd group (those with neurological signs) were more likely to suffer long term disability compared to those in groups 1 and 2a (without neck motion loss). However, these conclusions have been challenged by many as being too simple because they do not include the psychological problems like depression, anxiety, and poor coping abilities, all of which play an important role in predicting long term disability. Also, treatment strategies must include aspects to deal with the post-traumatic stress disorder, anxiety, depression and coping, not just the biological injury aspects. A convincing study published in 2008 looked at 226 studies on this subject and reported on 7 prognostic factors and found that 50-75% of people with current neck pain will report neck pain again 1-5 years later. Older age and psychosocial factors including psychological health, coping patterns, and the need to socialize were the strongest predictors. Three other potential predictors that require more investigation include the presence of arthritis, genetic factors, and compensation policies.

The bottom line or best advice to minimize our chances of having chronic, disabling neck pain after a car crash is, <u>don't stop living</u>! That is to say, carry on with work and hobbies as much as you possibly can so that you don't fall into the negative spiral of disability. If you feel yourself slipping, get help sooner than later! Pain relief and function restoration are strong goals and chiropractic has been found to be one of the first and most effective forms of treatment recommended by all treatment guidelines published on whiplash management.

Whiplash and Treatment Delay: Does it Matter?

When a person is involved in a car accident and has whiplash injuries, the inevitable question comes up: should I see a doctor? In most cases the answer is yes. But why is this important?

A car accident between two vehicles imparts a considerable amount of force on the body and spine. Even in low speed collisions, the forces add up to several times the force of gravity. So what does this mean? It means your body generally cannot resist such large forces without being injured. These whiplash injuries may be minor, such as a muscle strain or more substantial, involving stretching of the disks and ligaments of the spine.

Will these whiplash injuries always cause neck pain or headaches right after the collision? Only if there is severe damage to tissues will you experience immediate pain after a collision. In fact, having instant severe pain is a good indicator that you suffered a severe trauma. But most low speed collisions do not produce this type of instantaneous and intense pain. Instead, the person may feel "shaken up" or a little stiff. Unfortunately many patients interpret this stiffness as nothing more than a simple muscle strain and do not seek treatment for whiplash injuries. Up to two weeks can go by before you start to feel the effects of a whiplash injury. This is why it is important to see a doctor immediately to see if things are truly ok following an auto accident.

Only a doctor can examine your spine, pressing on different structures and seeing if your movements are fluid, pain-free and symmetrical. You will find it difficult to do this type of examination on yourself. In addition, x-rays may be needed to see the posture and alignment of your cervical spine. If you had radiating pain or symptoms of a brain injury, then an MRI may also be needed to see the soft tissues that x-rays cannot detect.

Without these types of important examinations it is hard to say if you've been injured significantly following an accident. Treatment delay, if you have been injured, will not help to get you back to health quickly. In fact, if you limited your activities and neck movements, this could impair your function down the road. Simply taking pain medications to restore the alignment of your spine will not be enough.

Minimizing Your Risk for Whiplash

While it is hard prevent someone from crashing their car into your car, there are some things you can do to minimize whiplash injuries.

The first preventive measure is making sure your seat is upright and the head rest touches the top of your head. If there is a lot of distance between your head and the rest, it will do little to help in the event of a collision. Also, if the headrest is too low, in can act as fulcrum, leveraging your neck into a worse position, and increasing injury risk.

Another thing we can do minimize injury risk is being in the best possible shape prior to the trauma. Research has shown people with good aerobic fitness seem to be more resilient after whiplash accidents.

If you are aware you are about to be hit, it is probably best to remain in a neutral position with eyes facing forward. People with their head turned prior to impact seem to have worse ligament injuries.

If you can afford it, a larger car will lessen the momentum of your vehicle after a collision. There are now vehicles with whiplash-protection seats (e.g. Saab) that dampen the effects of rear end-accidents. Frontal collisions tend to be less severe to the neck if the speeds are equal because the chin can hit the chest preventing forward motion of the neck. Rear-end and side-impact collisions do not have this benefit.

Unfortunately, there are many simply unavoidable risk factors. Women and children seem to be more vulnerable, possibly because of the increased head to neck size ratio. Also if you've ever had a head or neck trauma before and or have a degenerated disk in the neck, these factors elevate your risk for a more pronounced injury. Other factors that can slow your recovery include wearing a neck brace/collar, taking to bed rest, or getting vertical traction treatments. Inhibiting movements can feel good initially but is not good in the long term because of decreased muscle function and strength. Getting diagnosed as soon as possible can determine the best course of action for getting you to back to a speedy recovery. Just letting things go is rarely a good solution.

What Causes Whiplash?

The most common causes of "whiplash" are injuries that arise from automobile accidents or motor vehicle collisions (MVC's). So, let's chat about why and how this happens in a "typical" MVC. You are stopped at a red light, patiently waiting for the light to turn green and suddenly, you hear the screech of tires followed by a sudden jolt as the car from behind collides into the back of your vehicle.

By reflex, you may turn your head to the right to look in the rearview mirror to see what is happening. Even if you see the inevitable collision prior to the impact, the sudden jolt occurs so fast that you really don't have a chance to adequately brace and you feel yourself being forced back into the seat and headrest followed by a rebound forwards.

Since you always wear your seatbelt, you feel the restraint across your chest and lap belts tighten as you're propelled forward. The seat belt stops you from hitting the steering wheel or worse, propelling you forward through the windshield but by now, the damage has been done! This ALL occurs in less than 500 milliseconds – you cannot voluntarily contract your muscles this fast, which means even if you had time to prepare yourself for the impact by bracing, you can't stop the whiplash effect!

In a recent study, it was found the muscles in the front of the neck contract first at about 100 ms, which is 25 ms too late to prevent ligament or muscle damage, and they reach their peak stretch at 150ms (see 3rd from the left picture on the following page).

The muscles in the back of the neck start contracting soon thereafter but are injured more than the muscles in the front of the neck around the 300ms point. The reason for this is because as the head rebounds forwards, the muscles in the back of the neck are in the process of tightening up or shortening at the same time they are being stretched – NOT a good combination! This is one reason why many people injured in MVC's complain of neck pain greater in the back of the neck.

This also helps explain why headaches are common symptoms associated with whiplash as the upper 3 nerves that exit the top of the spine in the neck go into the head/scalp and are compressed or squeezed by the tight muscles in the back of the neck when they are injured which results in headaches.

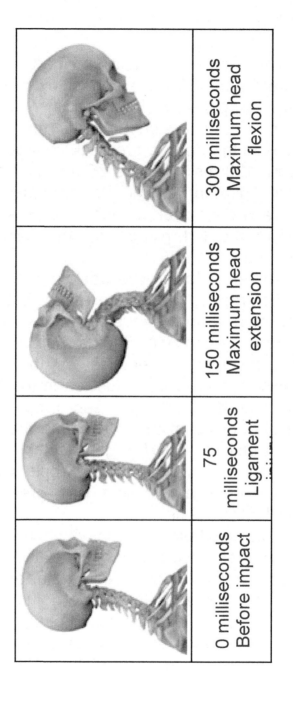

Whiplash-are you covered?

Americans are addicted to their automobiles. Nowhere else in the world do privately owned cars enjoy such an integrated connection to our everyday lives.

Many hours spent driving and in traffic do increase the possibility that one day an unfortunate accident will occur. Even if you are the best and most safe driver, this does little to keep someone else from hitting you.

Most states require insurance as a condition for the privilege of using the public roads and highways. But how much insurance should one carry? What does it cost to repair a car today, and perhaps more importantly, what does it cost to get you back to work and healthy again after a whiplash-type of trauma?

It may surprise you how much a ride in the ambulance, or a short stay in the hospital will set you back. Although chiropractic care expenses are generally less than care provided at hospitals or by surgeons, the costs can add up quickly, especially if you've suffered significant injury to your ligaments, disks and nerves after an auto accident in Las Vegas.

That's why it's important that you have adequate coverage should the unexpected occur. Periodically review your insurance coverage and make sure it is keeping up with the times. You don't want to be caught in a bind where your coverage does not meet your needs. In areas of insurance, med-pay and underinsured/not insured policies, help to protect you when others are not adequately covered and help to offset the costs of your treatment. Your insurance agent can help you navigate the various policy options that will best protect you and your family. Most agents will consult with you at no charge, so take advantage of their expertise.

And if you have suffered a whiplash injury, a doctor of chiropractic can properly assess the extent of spinal trauma and provide non-drug and non-surgical treatment for your neck, back or shoulder pain. Most whiplash injuries from auto accidents result in tears and sprain of the delicate ligaments that support the bones of the neck. Chiropractic doctors often specialize in the treatment of patients with spine and neck trauma after a car accident.

Whiplash Associated Disorders

Is the speed of a car crash directly proportional to amount of injury sustained to the occupants? One would expect more injury to occur when the speed of the collision is faster. Sometimes, this is the case – especially when car accidents occur at highway speeds.

However, what about the cases where a patient ends up in a lot of pain even when the speeds are quite slow, especially when there is little to no damage to the vehicle? , The answer to this seemingly paradoxical relationship has to do with plastic vs. elastic deformity.

This may be more simply understood if you think of "plastic" as something (in this case, your car) breaking apart vs. "elastic" as bouncing off without deforming or breaking apart. Therefore, in plastic deformity, there is more damage to the vehicle and in elastic deformity, there is little to no damage. When there is more metal crushing or more vehicular damage (plastic deformity), the G-forces associated with the crash are absorbed by the crushing metal, which in turn, exerts LESS G-forces to the contents inside the vehicle (i.e., the occupants), resulting in less injury. On the other hand, in the stiffer, less damaged vehicle, the energy is not absorbed by crushing metal (elastic deformity), resulting in the contents or occupants inside the vehicle being jostled or thrown about to a greater extent (due to the higher G-forces are exerted) and are at a greater risk for a higher degree of injury.

To illustrate this point, let's say that, we have a car that hits a solid brick wall at 10 mph that crushes in the front of the car 5 inches. In the second scenario, let's keep the car at a speed 10 mph, but because of a different car design (stiffer frame such as a solid bumper-to-bumper chassis), the crush in this instance is only 2 inches.

In the first example, the acceleration is found to be 8 G's of force. In the second example, acceleration is equals about 20 Gs of force. Thus, a collision with the same velocity, but with a crush amount smaller by 2.5 times will have a resulting G force 2.5 times larger.

Facts such as these are VERY important for you, your family and your doctor to appreciate, especially if there is legal action being taken in the case.

Therefore, it is important for you to choose a health care provider who understands and appreciates the potential impact this information carries when addressing your health related needs and communicating this information to others involved in a case.

Whiplash – What is the Best Type of Treatment?

Whiplash usually occurs when the head is suddenly whipped or snapped due to a sudden jolt, usually involving a motor vehicle collision. However, it can also occur from a slip and fall injury. So the question on deck is, which of the health care services best addresses the injured whiplash patient?

This question was investigated in a published study titled, A symptomatic classification of whiplash injury and the implications for treatment (*Journal of Orthopedic Medicine* 1999;21(1):22-25). The authors state conventional [medical] treatment utilized in whiplash care, "is disappointing." The authors' reference a study that demonstrated chiropractic treatment benefited 26 of 28 patients with chronic whiplash syndrome. The objective of their study was to determine which type of chronic whiplash patient would benefit the most from chiropractic treatment. They separated patients into one of 3 groups: **Group 1:** patients with "neck pain radiating in a 'coat hanger' distribution, associated with restricted range of neck movement but with no neurological deficit"; **Group 2:** patients with "neurological symptoms, signs or both in association with neck pain and a restricted range of neck movement"; **Group 3:** patients who described "severe neck pain but all of whom had a full range of motion and no neurological symptoms or signs distributed over specific myotomes or dermatomes." These patients also "described an unusual complex of symptoms," including "blackouts, visual disturbances, nausea, vomiting and chest pain, along with a nondermatomal distribution of pain."

The patients underwent an average of 19.3 adjustments over the course of 4.1 months (mean). The patients were then surveyed and their improvement was reported:

Group 1

38%	Asymptomatic
43%	Improved by Two Symptom Grades
13%	Improved by One Symptom Grade
6%	No Improvement

Group 2

24%	Asymptomatic
24%	Improved by Two Symptom Grades
24%	Improved by One Symptom Grade
28%	No Improvement

Group 3

0%	Asymptomatic
9%	Improved by Two Symptom Grades
18%	Improved by One Symptom Grade
64%	No Improvement
9%	Got Worse

These findings show the best chiropractic treatment results occur in patients with mechanical neck pain (group 1) and / or those with neurological losses (group 2). The exaggerated group (group 3) was the most challenging and, the only group where a small percentage worsened. The good news is, the number of cases that responded well to chiropractic treatment (groups 1 & 2) far outnumber those that don't (group 3). **Hence, most patients with whiplash injuries should consider chiropractic as their first choice of health care provision.**

Interesting Facts about Whiplash

We all know the most common causes of "whiplash" are injuries that typically arise from automobile accidents or, motor vehicle collisions (MVC's) although whiplash can also occur from slip and fall and virtually, any injury where your head is whipped backwards. But there are many things about whiplash you may not be aware of, which is the reason for this month's Heath Update on whiplash.

For example, did you know the effect whiplash has on public health (in general) is tremendous? The number of cases occurring annually is frequently quoted as 1,000,000 per year, but this is based on an outdated (1971) and incomplete dataset. A more recent figure of 3 million per year is considered to be more accurate because it's based on several governmental databases and it accounts for the expected number of unreported cases by the NHTSA (National Highway Traffic Safety Administration). That's a huge difference! The updated figure accounts for whiplash victims not attended to by emergency medical services. In less catastrophic accidents, the injured party may not appear to be significantly injured at the scene of the MVC and decline emergency care and hence, the MVC will to unreported to a governmental data collection center.

Another interesting study surveyed over 3500 chiropractors who were asked if they commonly applied cervical (neck) spinal manipulation to patients who had known herniated or protruded disks (in their neck). Over 90% of the chiropractors indicated they found it safe and effective to utilize cervical adjustments (manipulation) in this patient population. It is VERY important for you to know this as frequently, you may be told by your medical doctor (or next door neighbor), "...don't let anyone crack your neck!" Now, you can rest assured that in the experience of MANY chiropractors (not just me), significant benefits can be achieved by this treatment approach. Moreover, the sooner neck adjustments are applied, the better the results - so don't wait to get a chiropractic treatment after an MVC!

Another interesting study investigated the "proper" or "best" seated position in a car during a rear-end collision, based on an analysis of many previously published studies on this topic. Because the seated position of the person involved in a MVC is related to the degree of the injury, the factors studied included the angle of the seat back, seat-bottom angle, the density of the foam in the seatback, the height above the floor [of the knees], and the presence of armrests in cars. They found that the seat back angle of 110-130 degrees reduced disk pressure and low back muscle activity but 110 degrees – MAX. – was found to minimize the forward positioning of the head. A 5 degree downwards tilt of the seat bottom further reduced the pressure in the low back disks and muscle activity as measured by EMG (electromyography). The use of armrests and the use of a lumbar support were also found to be important to reduce injuries associated with MVCs. This combination was reported to be optimum for all of us to use in order to minimize the bodily injury in a rear-end MVC. Other important factors included firm dense foam in the seat back, an adjustable seat bottom (for angle, height, and front to back distance), horizontal & vertical lumbar support adjustments (…best if they pulsate to reduce the static load encountered in a crash), seat shock absorbers, and seat adjustments for front to back to adjust for different patient heights.

Whiplash and Your Ligaments

Most people who get a whiplash-like injury think it is caused by a problem in their muscles. It's easy to see this why this may be the case since muscle pain following car accidents is so common. Deep pain and even spasm can occur after severe trauma resulting in daily pain and even headaches. Since our 10-12 pound head is attached to our necks, by muscles that go into the shoulder region, whiplash injuries after a car accident can feel like a muscle pull and taking muscle relaxants seems a reasonable approach.

Although tears of muscles fibers do occur in whiplash injuries, these can heal rather quickly due to the rich blood supply. The ligaments such as disks hold the joints of the neck together keeping the nerves from being pressed upon and stretched. These are the structures that are critically injured during whiplash injuries. The muscles that contract to protect the joints from moving too much are generally less of a problem than when the ligaments are injured. A recent study (BMC Musculoskeletal Discord 2006;21:103) showed that after a whiplash injury, the strength of the neck ligaments is further reduced. This means that you are more susceptible to getting injured if you previously suffered a trauma.

To detect ligament injuries you can look at MRIs immediately after the trauma. In many cases they can show small tears or the inflammation and swelling that goes with tears of these important structures.

You can also have stress x-rays taken in the positions of forward and backward bending. These types of x-rays can show which ligaments have been traumatized and are allowing the bones of the neck to move too much. When this increased motion is severe, this is called instability. Some newer MRI machines can scan in different positions so that the tears and their motion effects are seen with one test. Some people may find the MRI scanner to be a bit restrictive or claustrophobic. X-rays are usually the most practical and least costly choice.

Whiplash! Do I Need an Attorney?

When you hear the word, "whiplash," it brings to mind many different thoughts – motor vehicle collision (MVC), neck pain, headaches, concussion, jaw pain, litigation, car damage estimates – possibly a new car, medical costs, doctor's appointments, sleepless nights, and more. Questions typically asked when a MVC occurs include the following: 1. Do I need to get an attorney? 2. What can I expect for recovery time from my neck pain? 3. Why is it taking so long to get my car fixed? 4. Should I talk to the insurance company when they call? 5. I have to give a deposition next week. What is that? 6. My case didn't settle and we're going to court. How do I prepare for that? 7. The insurance company is offering $XXXX.XX for a settlement. What do you think my problems will be down the road?

Let's take a look at these!

- Should you obtain the services of an attorney? If you want to significantly reduce your stress when it comes time to negotiating with the insurance company, especially towards the end of the process, then YES! Needless to say, you HAVE

TO seek council if you plan to not settle and need to go to court. However, you do not have to get an attorney immediately unless you just don't want to deal with the insurance company at all. Typically, it's worth having an attorney as they are experienced in "…the process."
- Recovery from neck pain can vary between a simple strain at 6-8 weeks to a herniated disk that may require surgery. We recommend you ask us this question about once a month as it will help you decide about this as well as questions 1 and 7.
- The insurance company may delay the payment of the car repair costs for a number of reasons. Until the insurance company inspects the car's damages, they will not authorize the repair shop work, which can take weeks!
- If you have hired an attorney, he/she will communicate for you. If not, it is appropriate for you to communicate with the insurance company. The important thing is to NOT settle the claim until you're sure you can do all of your pre-MVC activities without difficulty or pain, which often can take a full year or more.
- These are call "discovery depositions" where you will be asked questions about the accident such as, where you hurt,

what you can and can't do since the MVC, what tests and treatment you've received and what the results were. Your attorney will tell you the strengths and weaknesses of your case. The deposition "process" is quite easy and there is no reason to feel intimidated. Most attorneys are very courteous and will treat you kindly so don't worry unnecessarily!
- Preparing for court is similar except you can't ask questions – they ask & you answer! Your attorney will tell you to answer only the question being asked and your attorney will later be able to ask you to clarify what was "left out." Always be kind, courteous, and NEVER let the other attorney get you angry!
- See #2 above. If you have ongoing radiating pain in your arm (from your neck) or leg (from your low back), the "prognosis" for complete recovery is less favorable. Similarly, if you have ligament damage in your neck, there will probably be an accelerated pace of arthritis formation that may not bother you much for 5-10 years or longer but may later in life. We, as your expert witness, will describe your "impairment" and bring this to the jury's attention.

The Whiplash Syndrome

The term "whiplash" was coined by Dr. Harold Crowe in 1928 during an interview on car collision related neck injuries but he reportedly "...regretted it later." The term "whiplash" quickly became a household word and relates to a sudden movement of the head producing a neck sprain. It is now accepted that not only forward/backward movements during motor vehicle collisions (MCV) result in neck injury but also side to side and angular movements at the time of impact. In the past, we've discussed the number of milliseconds that takes place during the whiplash process after impact (~500 msec.) and the fact that voluntary muscle contraction takes longer (~800 msec.) making it next to impossible to adequately "brace" prior to impact, even when the collision is anticipated. Today, we're going to look at the symptoms and complaints that are commonly described by whiplash patients.

"Early whiplash syndrome" is defined as the condition where immediate or very close to immediate symptoms are noted. One study reported symptoms commonly described after a MVC include the following: neck pain (93%), headache (72%), shoulder pain (49%) and back pain (38%) and, 87% of patients had multiple symptoms. Others reported nausea (48%) and dizziness (38%) as initial symptoms. For some, many of these symptoms resolve within days, weeks or months leaving a smaller percentage with symptoms that last beyond 6 months, which is then referred to as "late whiplash syndrome." In one study of 52 patients, symptoms improved over a 2 week to 12 month time frame but then remained static or unchanged for the following year. Another study of 117 patients at the 2-year point, reported the following symptoms (the frequency of occurrence is in parentheses): Neck pain (17%), headache (15%), fatigue (13%), shoulder pain (13%), insomnia (12%), anxiety (11%), concentration loss (10%), and forgetfulness (10%).

Reasons for the continuation into a late syndrome are supported by two possible causes. 1. It is due to a high level initial symptom, including severe neck pain and headache often with radiating arm pain (radiculopathy). 2. It is caused by the stressful events that are present either at the time of the motor vehicle collision or soon thereafter. These stressors could include work loss, marital stress, financial stress, and/or depression or anxiety issues associated with being injured. It was also reported that the specific type of headache suffered in the late whiplash syndrome in a 47 patient study, 74% had tension-type headache, 15% had migraine and 11% had cervicogenic headache. Some authors have reported that the type of headaches that occur as a result of an MVC are similar to almost identical to those seen after head trauma from other causes including sports injuries such as football, hockey, and boxing.

Because "whiplash" results in a mechanical type of injury to the small joints of the neck, muscles and ligaments, the only logical choice for management and treatment is chiropractic. This is because chiropractic addresses the mechanical injury with a manual, hands-on approach specifically aimed at restoring function in the injured area. Studies are clear that whiplash patients make a faster, less painful recovery, return to work and desired activities faster and are the most satisfied when utilizing chiropractic when compared to covering up the symptoms with medications that have negative side effects that interfere with being able to think and ultimately, reduce productivity.

Mild Traumatic Brain Injury – What's That?

When you woke up today, you thought this was like any other Tuesday. You packed the kid's lunches and off to school they went. You're on your way to work and everything is on schedule- it's a good day! You are stopped at a red light when out of nowhere, someone crashes into the back end of your car and you feel your head snap back over the headrest and then bounce forwards, almost hitting the steering with your forehead. Everything goes blank for a second or two. "What just happened?" Initially, you're in "shock," and after checking to make sure you're not bleeding, you notice that your neck and head are hurting in a way that's new to you. When the police arrive and start asking you questions about what had happened, you try to piece together the sequence of events of the collision but you're not quite sure how it all fits together. Your memory just isn't real clear. Within the first few days, significant neck pain and headache overshadow everything else but you begin to notice that you're ability to "think clearly" is just not quite right. Your memory seems fuzzy, you lose your train of thought easily, sometimes in the middle of a discussion, and you are tired – really tired! Taking a nap several times a day is needed. The other day, you were discussing a project with a group of co-workers and you had to ask "...now where was I?" several times during the discussion as you lost your place in the middle of a thought.

Mild traumatic brain injury or, MTBI, is exactly what is described above. Many patients do not even mention these things to their chiropractor when they present after a car crash as it's hard to describe these symptoms and many feel it's just because they are tired or upset about the accident. When directly asked if any of these symptoms exist, the patient is often surprised and say, "...how did you know?" They are even more surprised when they learn there is an actual reason and explanation for feeling this way. Most of the time, the patient has to be asked if these symptoms exist! This is actually "normal" behavior for those suffering from MTBI.

To better understand how this occurs, think of the more catastrophic situation where the person hits their head to the point of creating an internal bleed and is unconscious. In this case, it's easier to appreciate the presence of a "brain injury." With severe head trauma, the person usually has significant memory loss, having no memory of the accident and maybe worse, not being able to recognize family or friends. Losing the memory of days, weeks, months or years of time is common with these severe head injuries. However, in MTBI, there is less bruising to the brain and consequently, there are less severe symptoms. Though the symptoms are similar, MTBI is in a way, a mild form of the above. With MTBI, the person does NOT have to hit their head on anything to bruise the brain. This is because the speed at which the head is propelled forward and back literally slams the brain into the inside walls, creating the bruising. Because the brain is suspended inside our skull, damage to some of the nerve cells occurs, most commonly the brain stem, the frontal lobe and/or the temporal lobe.

Depending on which part of the brain is injured, the physical findings may include problems with walking, balance, coordination, strength/endurance, as well as difficulties with communicating ("cognitive deficits"), processing information, memory, and altered psychological functions. Recognizing these symptoms and managing MTBI in a coordinated approach with a neuropsychologist is sometimes needed.

The Whiplash Syndrome: Ringing in the Ears

The term "whiplash" usually brings to mind neck pain, headaches and/or a stiff neck. However, there are other symptoms associated with whiplash that we don't usually think of, such as ringing in the ears or, tinnitus. In the absence of whiplash, there are many people who experience an occasional ringing or sound of some sort in their ears. The ringing may seem to keep time with the heartbeat or, in cadence with breathing and is more common over the age of 40, and more common in men. The sound can be a buzzing, ringing, roaring, hissing or high pitched noise that usually lasts only seconds or minutes at the most. So, think of those times when you've noticed tinnitus and ask yourself, "...how would that affect me if that noise never stopped or lasted for hours?"

Before we discuss the association of tinnitus with whiplash, let's review some facts about tinnitus. There are two primary types of tinnitus: Pulsatile and Nonpulsatile. Pulsatile tinnitus is often caused by sounds created either by blood flow problems in the face or neck, muscle movements near the ear, or changes in the ear canal. The nonpulsatile tinnitus is usually caused by nerve problems involving hearing in one or both ears. The later is sometimes described as a sound coming from inside the head. The most common cause of tinnitus is from hearing loss that occurs from aging – technically called presbycusis. However, it can also occur from living or working in a loud environment. Tinnitus can occur with many types of hearing loss and can be a symptom of almost any ear disorder. Other common causes include earwax buildup, certain medication side effects (aspirin, antibiotics), too much caffeine or alcohol intake, ear infections – which can lead to rupture of the eardrum, dental problems, TMJ or jaw problems, following surgery or radiation therapy to the head or neck, a rapid change in environmental pressure (airplane rides, elevators, scuba diving), severe weight loss from malnutrition or dieting, bicycle riding with the neck extended for lengthy timeframes, high blood pressure, nerve conditions (MS, migraine headache), as well as other conditions such as acoustic neuroma, anemia, labyrinthitis, Meniere's disease, otosclerosis and thyroid disease. The good news is that most of the time, tinnitus comes and goes and does not require treatment. When tinnitus is associated with other symptoms, does not get better or go away, or is in only one ear, it is wise to consult with us. Spinal manipulation and other chiropractic treatment approaches are often VERY helpful in resolving tinnitus with the benefits of avoiding the need for medications, all of which carry secondary side effects. Chiropractic approaches are also highly effective when tinnitus is accompanied by dizziness or vertigo, usually requiring treatment applied to the upper neck area.

So, how does whiplash cause tinnitus? There are primary as well as secondary causes that can give rise to tinnitus after whiplash. After looking at the long list of causes above, direct trauma to the head such as hitting the side window, the back of the seat, the steering wheel, mirror and/or windshield makes obvious sense. Secondary causes often involve the TMJ or jaw which is commonly injured in whiplash. By itself, TMJ can cause ear pain, tinnitus, vertigo (dizziness), hearing loss, and headaches. Because many nerves that innervate the neck and head arise from the neck as well as from the cranial nerves, spinal manipulation of the neck as well as certain cranial manipulations can have a dramatic benefit in treatment of whiplash induced tinnitus.

What Really Causes Whiplash?

Whiplash is a non-medical term for a condition that occurs when the neck and head move rapidly forwards and backwards or, sideways, at a speed so fast our neck muscles are unable to stop the movement from happening. This sudden force results in the normal range of motion being exceeded and causes injury to the soft tissues (muscles, tendons and ligaments) of the neck. Classically, whiplash is associated with car accidents or, motor vehicle collisions (MVCs) but can also be caused by other injuries such as a fall on the ice and banging the head, sports injuries, as well as being assaulted, including "shaken baby syndrome."

The History of Whiplash. The term "Whiplash" was first coined in 1928 when pilots were injured by landing airplanes on air craft carriers in the ocean. Their heads were snapped forwards and back as they came to a sudden stop. There are many synonyms for the term "whiplash" including, but not limited to, cervical hyperextension injury, acceleration-deceleration syndrome, cervical sprain (meaning ligament injury) and cervical strain (meaning muscle / tendon injury). In spite of this, the term "whiplash" has continued to be used usually in reference to MVCs.

Why Whiplash Occurs. As noted previously, we cannot voluntarily stop our head from moving beyond the normal range of motion as it takes only about 500 milliseconds for whiplash to occur during a MVC, and we cannot voluntarily contract our neck muscles in less than 800-1000 msec. The confusing part about whiplash is that it can occur in low speed collisions such as 5-10 mph, sometimes more often than at speeds of 20 mph or more. The reason for this has to do with the vehicle absorbing the energy of the collision. At lower speeds, there is less crushing of the metal (less damage to the vehicle) and therefore, less of the energy from the collision is absorbed. The energy from the impact is then transferred to the contents inside the vehicle (that is, you)! This is technically called elastic deformity – when there is less damage to the car, more energy is transferred to the contents inside the car. When metal crushes, energy is absorbed and less energy affects the vehicle's contents (technically called plastic deformity). This is exemplified by race cars. When they crash, they are made to break apart so the contents (the driver) is less jostled by the force of the collision. Sometimes, all that is left after the collision is the cage surrounding the driver.

Whiplash Symptoms. Symptoms can occur immediately or within minutes to hours after the initial injury. Also, less injured areas may be overshadowed initially by more seriously injured areas and may only "surface" after the more serious injured areas improve. The most common symptoms include neck pain, headaches, and limited neck movement (stiffness). Neck pain may radiate into the middle back area and/or down an arm. If arm pain is present, a pinched nerve is a distinct possibility. Also, mild brain injury can occur even when the head is not bumped or hit. These symptoms include difficulty staying on task, losing your place in the middle of thought or sentences and tiredness/fatigue. These symptoms often resolve within 6 weeks with a 40% chance of still hurting after 3 months, and 18% chance after 2 years. There is no reliable method to predict the outcome. Studies have shown that early mobilization and manipulation results in a better outcome than waiting for weeks or months to seek chiropractic treatment. The best results are found by obtaining prompt evaluation for chiropractic care.

More Whiplash Facts

Whiplash is a fairly common condition that occurs when the neck is suddenly forced forwards and backwards, usually from motor vehicle collisions. Before 1928, whiplash was sometimes called "railway spine" as it was used to describe injuries that occurred to people involved in train accidents. Since 1928, much has been studied and reported about this condition and in 1995, the term, "whiplash associated disorders" or WAD, was introduced. The WAD classification of whiplash patients includes 3 main category (WAD I, II and III) and a few years later, WAD II was broken into 2 sub-categories (WAD I, IIa, IIb, III). This occurred because some patients in WAD II took a longer time to heal than others. Here are the basic definitions of WAD I, II, III:

- WAD I: Patients have complaints but no objective findings meaning we cannot reproduce your pain during our examinations
- WAD IIa: Patients have complaints with objective findings but a normal range of movement of the neck and no neurological findings (normal strength and sensation ability)

- WAD IIb: Same as WAD IIa except here, neck movements are decreased
- WAD III: Here, neurological abnormal findings (weakness and/or sensation) are present.
- WAD IV: Includes fractures and dislocations. Because of this unique difference, this category is often left out of the research that uses this category system to determine prognosis of the WAD case.

This system is very useful as it has the ability to predict the results in a case long before the conclusion of the case.

We have discussed the cause of whiplash in previous articles and what happens when we are hit from behind unexpectedly. In essence, we cannot guard against the abnormal forces that occur in the neck as it all happens faster than we can voluntarily contract our muscles. Also, the myth about no car damage = no injury is just that – a myth! In fact, in low speed impacts, less damage to the car transfers greater forces to the contents inside because the energy of the force is not absorbed by crushing metal (elastic vs. plastic deformity).

Symptoms of whiplash vary widely. Most common symptoms include neck pain and stiffness, headache, shoulder pain/stiffness, dizziness, fatigue, jaw pain, arm pain, arm weakness, visual disturbances, ringing ear noises, and sometimes back pain. If symptoms continue and chronic WAD occurs, depression, anger, frustration, anxiety, stress, drug dependency, post-traumatic stress syndrome, sleep disturbance, and social isolation can occur.

Diagnosis is based on the history, physical exam, x-ray, MRI, and if nerve damage occurs (WAD III), an EMG. Treatment includes rest, ice and later heat, exercise, pain management and avoiding prolonged use of a collar. Chiropractic includes all of these as well as manipulation, mobilization, muscle release methods, and patient education. Prompt return to normal activity including work is important to avoid the negative spiral into long term disability.

Whiplash: Can It Be Prevented?

Whiplash, or cervical acceleration-deceleration disorder (CAD) often occurs in car collisions. So, the question is raised, "...can it be prevented?" To answer this we must first consider the obvious facts about minimizing your distractions when you drive: intoxication, engaged conversation (especially if you're trying to make eye contact), talking on your cell phone or worse, texting while driving (equal to 3 mixed drinks!!!), messing with the radio, GPS, or other "gadgets" in the car, eating while driving, putting on makeup, shaving, and yes, even reading a book while driving! If you're getting tired pull over for a "power nap." Even a 15-20 min. "shut eye" session can really help. But these things are obvious (and WELL DOCUMENTED)! What other factors, like features in cars can minimize or possibly prevent injury in the event of a crash?

The headrest is a very most important feature in the vehicle for preventing or at least reducing the degree of injury in a crash. Unfortunately, most people do not bother setting the headrest at the correct height, as it's usually in a position that is too low. When this occurs, the head can slide over the top of the headrest which can actually result in greater injury as it acts like a fulcrum allowing the head to hyperextend over it. It can also make the injuries associated with whiplash much worse. The proper height of the headrest should be no lower than the top of the ear level but in a lot of cases, the top third of the head may be a better choice, especially if the headrest is small in size or, if the seat is reclined. The angle of the seatback is important with reference to headrests because when the seatback is reclined, there is a certain amount of "ramping" that occurs in rear-end collisions. This is because when the seat is reclined back, the seatback can act literally like a ramp and your whole body can slide up the ramp/seatback and your head can end up over the top of headrest. Therefore, keep the seatback as vertical as you can tolerate. The degree of "spring" or bounce of the seat back also affects the speed or acceleration of the rebound that occurs in a crash but unfortunately, the seat's "springiness" can't really be changed.

      Seat belts and airbags are a great pair of safety features as they work together to reduce the chances of a serious injury, as well as whiplash. The seatbelt's job is to stabilize the trunk and prevent the occupant from being ejected from the vehicle while the airbag protects the chest, neck and head from hitting the steering wheel or windshield. Seatbelts arrived on the scene in the 1970s, shoulder restraints shortly thereafter, and airbags in 1985. An 8 year study by the U of Pittsburgh reported on over 7000 spine injured patients, and found a significant reduction of spine related injuries when both seatbelts and airbags were utilized. The National Highway Traffic Safety Administration advises at least a 10-inch distance between the steering wheel and the breastbone in order to avoid airbag injuries, which reportedly occur within the first 2-3 inches of the airbag.

The "take home" message here is when you combine: 1. Staying alert by avoiding all the many distractions that can lure your eyes off the road; 2. Slowing down when you see or sense trouble, and, 3. Making sure your seatbelt is fastened (and those of your passengers, as well) and your airbag still works, you can be quite confident you are doing your part in preventing injury (including whiplash) for both yourself and potentially others!

Whiplash - Biomechanics and Costs

Whiplash or Cervical Acceleration-deceleration Disorder (CAD) is primarily associated with motor vehicle collisions (MVCs) and in particular, rear-end collisions. Last month, we discussed how CAD can be prevented and focused greatly on paying attention while driving and, the position of the headrest. Whiplash is defined as an injury to the cervical spine (neck) caused by a rapid/sudden, usually unexpected, forceful movement. (Typically, forwards and backwards, if struck from in front or behind, or, a side to side movement if struck from the side.) Even worse, when coupled with the head being rotated at the time of impact, tearing of the ligaments, muscles, and joint capsules in the neck can cause a myriad of symptoms that can remain present for years, sometimes permanently. Some of these symptoms include:

- Neck and shoulder pain and/or stiffness
- Middle and low back pain
- Dizziness
- Vertigo (balance disturbance)
- Fatigue
- Numbness/Tingling

- Face/Jaw pain
- Cognitive dysfunction or brain injury (even without hitting the head directly)
- Sleep disorders

A report published in January 2011 discussed recent advances and a new law that goes into effect 9-1-11 regarding the design of head restraints that is aimed at significantly reducing the injury severity and consequently the costs associated with CAD. The Code of Regulations (CFR) describes the new bill, (FMVSS 202a) as a standard, "...to reduce the frequency and severity of neck injury in rear-end and other collisions." This new law requires testing the absorbency (springiness), the locking mechanisms, and the height by making sure the restraint is above the center of gravity of the occupant's head to reduce the "backset" (distance between the head and the restraint). This is done by testing the seat back and head restraint as a system to ensure the head restraint remains in its proper position throughout the collision. The concept is to reduce the rearward shift of the occupant's head relative to their torso or to avoid extreme hyperextension. Companies have been manufacturing both dynamic, as well as static, head restraint systems in response to this new requirement that becomes fully effective on 9-1-11 for both front and rear seats. So, how does this equate to costs?

Between the years of 1988 and 1996 from 805,851 whiplash injuries, the National Accident Sampling System (NASS) reported the total annual cost of treatment, excluding damage to property, was $5.2 billion. This amount includes costs derived from medical, legal, insurance, productivity loss and work loss. The report estimates, by improving the seat back and head restraint position to the occupant's head, a total reduction of 14,247 whiplash injuries is expected which will have a nearly $92 million total cost reduction through both direct injury costs and also the indirect societal costs!

Whiplash - Who Will Recover?

Whiplash, or Whiplash Associated Disorders (WAD), involves a cluster of symptoms and findings that include biomechanical or tissue injury findings, as well as psychological factors that accompany pain and disability. To answer the presenting question, who will recover from whiplash, a task force was set up to investigate this and research over a 10 year time frame was reviewed. They found the initial level of pain after the injury and the associated psychological factors are the two best predictors of whiplash recovery.

WAD results from a neck injury caused by a sudden back and forth movement of the head that often occurs during a car crash. The injury occurs because of the fact that the sudden movement happens in a shorter time frame than our ability to voluntarily contract our own neck muscles. Hence, even if we brace ourselves before the impact, we cannot avoid the sudden "crack the whip" phenomenon that occurs during a crash. It's even worse is if the head is turned at the time of impact! Although most WAD sufferers recover within a few months, many report ongoing pain a year or more later. With about 2 million insurance claims registered per year in the US, the focus is shifting from what causes pain to what recovery predictors exist with the focus on managing those that are manageable.

One of the two predictors reported was the level of pain reported by the patient 3 weeks after a motor vehicle collision (MVC). In a group of over 3000 patients with WAD, this was reported to be, "...the single most important predictor of who recovers in a timely manner." On a 10-point pain scale (10 being the most intense pain), patients with a score under 5 recovered more quickly.

The second of the two strong predictors was the patient's belief or expectation of recovery. Again, at the 3 week mark following the crash, over 1000 WAD injured patients were asked how likely they felt they would recover fully and at 6 months, the disability level was compared to those expectations gathered at the 3 week point. They found a 4x greater chance of being placed in a "more disabled" group if at the 3 week point, the patient reported a poor outcome expectation for recovery. Those who were reportedly prone to "catastrophic thinking" also fared poorly. These are the patients who can't stop focusing on pain – they believe the crash was, "...the worst thing that has ever happened to them."

They also found patients wearing a neck collar to protect and immobilize the neck following a MVC were no better off compared to those not wearing a collar. In fact, in one group of patients, those who wore the collar were absent longer from work and utilized more pain killing medications compared to those who did not wear it.

Whiplash - Which Treatment Method Is Best?

Whiplash, or better termed, cervical acceleration-deceleration disorder (CAD) is primarily an injury to the soft tissues of the neck – that is, the muscles, their tendon insertions, and the ligaments that hold the joints firmly together. Neck pain is a very common health problem that affects between 10–15% of the population and drives people to all types of health care providers. We have previously discussed the reasons why whiplash /CAD injuries occur, the examination process and the prognosis aspects but the argument continues as to what treatment methods work the best when managing patients with CAD.

In the May 21, 2002 issue of the Annals of Internal Medicine, a group of medical doctors and PhD's reported on neck pain treatment comparing traditional medical and physical therapy approaches verses spinal manipulation. In the study, they compared three common neck pain treatment approaches in a group of 183 patients with chronic neck pain (patients who had neck pain for more than 3 months). The 3 methods included traditional medical care which included medication utilization and rest, manual therapy (chiropractic adjustments) and physical therapy (active exercise training). After 7 weeks of treatment, the percentage of patients who felt either totally resolved (cured) or much improved were 68.3% receiving manual therapy / chiropractic care, 50.8% receiving physical therapy, and 35.9% receiving medical care. The author, Jan Lucas Hoving, PhD reports that manual therapy / chiropractic was found to be more effective than the other 2 methods "...on almost all outcome measures," not just a few! Further, although PT scored better than traditional medical care, "...most of the differences were not statistically significant," meaning, not that much better. The authors appropriately reported that further study was needed to better understand the differences between methods.

In 2008, the "Decade Task Force" reviewed 10 years of studies on the treatment of neck pain and found similar results and referenced many studies that indicated spinal manipulation for neck pain, headaches, whiplash, and other neck related conditions was one of the most effective methods and that patients with neck pain should be given the option of receiving manual therapy / chiropractic before other approaches as it was found to be less expensive, faster in obtaining satisfying results (shorter course of disability), and most effective in terms of long-term benefits.

This comparison discussion is by no means meant to minimize the importance of medical and PT care. However, there appears to be a bias among patients with neck pain to seek medical care first when the studies clearly show chiropractic care is the preferred method. Hence, the purpose of this article is to educate the reader that their choice in treatment for neck pain should favor chiropractic care FIRST, not last. In fact, the sooner manipulation can be applied to the injured joints of the neck, typically the faster the results. For example, long term disability and chronic neck pain can occur from prolonged use of a cervical collar as the structures tighten and stiffen up from being immobile - unable to move because of the collar. Unless there is some unstable condition to the neck (fracture, grade 3 ligament tear, progressive neurological loss, etc.), studies support manipulation / early mobilization of the neck joints after injuries like whiplash verses wearing a cervical collar and rest.

Car Accidents and Mild Traumatic Brain Injury

When you woke up today, you thought this was like any other Friday. You're on your way to work, and traffic is flowing smoother than normal. Suddenly, someone crashes into the back end of your car and you feel your head extend back over the headrest and then rebound forwards, almost hitting the steering with your forehead. It all happened so fast. After a few minutes, you notice your neck and head starting to hurt in a way you've not previously felt. When the police arrive and start asking questions about what had happened, you try to piece together what happened but you're not quite sure of the sequence of events. Your memory just isn't that clear. Within the first few days, in addition to significant neck and headache pain, you notice your memory seems fuzzy, and you easily lose your train of thought. Everything seems like an effort and you notice you're quite irritable. When your chiropractor asks you if you've felt any of these symptoms, you look at them and say, "...how did you know? I just thought I was having a bad day – I didn't know whiplash could cause these symptoms!"

Because these symptoms are often subtle and non-specific, it's quite normal for patients not to complain about them. In fact, we almost always have to describe the symptoms and ask if any of these symptoms "sound familiar" to the patient.

As pointed out above, patients with Mild Traumatic Brain Injury (MTBI) don't mention any of the previously described symptoms and in fact, may be embarrassed to discuss these symptoms with their chiropractor or physician when they first present after a car crash. This is because the symptoms are vague and hard to describe and, many feel the symptoms are caused by simply being tired or perhaps upset about the accident. When directly asked if any of these symptoms exist, the patient is often surprised there is an actual reason for feeling this way.

The cause of MTBI is due to the brain actually bouncing or rebounding off the inner walls of the bony skull during the "whiplash" process, when the head is forced back and forth after the impact. During that process, the brain which is suspended inside our skull, is forced forwards and literally ricochets off the skull and damages some of the nerve cells most commonly of either the brain stem (the part connected to the spinal cord), the frontal lobe (the part behind the forehead) and/or the temporal lobe (the part of the brain located on the side of the head).

Depending on the direction and degree of force generated by the collision (front end, side impact or rear end collision), the area of the brain that may be damaged varies as it could be the area closest to initial impact or, the area on the opposite side, due to the rebound effect. Depending on which part of the brain is injured, the physical findings may include problems with walking, balance, coordination, strength/endurance, as well as difficulties with communicating ("cognitive deficits"), processing information, memory, and altered psychological functions.

The good news is that most of these injuries will recover within 3-12 months but unfortunately, not all do and in these cases, the term, "post-concussive syndrome" is sometimes used.

Whiplash and Vision - What's The Connection?

In whiplash, "post concussive syndrome" (PCS) can affect up to 20-30% of patients who have had a mild head injury with resulting left over, long-term problems. Interestingly, eye movements have a close relationship to the function of the brain and can be an accurate measure for determining the presence of PCS as well as a good barometer for tracking the recovery process.

The correlation between eye movement and PCS was studied by a group of New Zealand researchers using 2 groups of 36 patients each – those with PCS who showed good recovery vs. those who did not at a 3-5 month point after their accident. The method of evaluating this included neuropsychological evaluations using various tools that assess memory, reading, recall, use of numbers, and other brain function tests.

They found the worse PCS patient group had poorer brain function test results and the correspondingly worse eye movement tests. Most interesting was that the group who had a better psychological recovery, STILL HAD eye movement abnormalities. This suggested, in spite of seemingly good recovery, injury to the brain persisted. They also stressed importance of the correlation between the psychological tests abnormalities now have a specific biological marker which can be used as a clinical "tool" and, that PCS is NOT merely a psychological condition.

PCS symptoms include headaches, dizziness, poor concentration, memory loss, irritability, mood swings and these and other symptoms vary between patients with PCS. This makes the assessment process challenging since each patient is rather unique in how PCS portrays itself. To make this more challenging, these symptoms can last for the first few hours after a motor vehicle collision with a mild closed head injury to days, weeks, months and even years after the injury, some with complete loss work capabilities and significant life impact.

The World Health Organization first clinically recognized PCS in 1992, with the American Psychiatric following in 1994. Another diagnostic challenge is that the conventional tests such as CT scans and MRI scans usually do not display abnormalities in most patients with PCS, thus doctors must rely on psychological tests to establish the diagnosis and track recovery (or lack thereof). More recently, special tests such as functional MRI, diffusion tensor imaging, MR spectroscopy and arterial spin labeling can help detect functional, structural, or perfusion changes in the brain but these tests are costly and not routinely available in most clinical settings.

There are also criticisms that these less available/costly tests can't track changes in function very well. Similarly, there exists criticism of neuropsychological test results being affected by uncontrollable factors such as age, education, state of employment, economic status, depression, malingering, and litigation.

The good news is that most patients with PCS largely resolve by 1-3 months post-injury. However, this reported rate of recovery relies on neuropsychological tests, which loses their ability to detect PCS with the passage of time.

The benefits of being able to detect brain injury which include complex reflex pathways and different parts of the brain through the measurement of eye movement is very important as no other method has yet been found to be as accurate and, is completely independent of intellectual ability and neuropsychological injury. The ability for eye movements to show abnormality at 3-5 months post-injury is tremendous!

Even More Whiplash Facts

In whiplash research, many articles have been published that conflict or contradict each other. The goal of this Health Update is to report the "facts" about whiplash.

- It is more common to have a delay in the onset of whiplash symptoms. Symptoms may start about two hours after the initial injury or it may take days, weeks, or months before you feel anything.
- For whiplash caused by car accidents, the severity depends on the force of the impact, the way you were seated in your car, and if you were properly restrained using a shoulder and seat belt.
- Tests show the soft tissues in your neck sustain injury at a threshold of 5 mph. That means if you're rear-ended at 5 mph or slower, you have a lower chance of getting whiplash. However, most rear-end car accidents happen at speeds of 6-12 mph.
- If you've been in a car accident, it's a good idea to be evaluated even if your car didn't get damaged and you don't feel any pain.

- Although whiplash is most often associated with car accidents, you can also get whiplash from sports such as snowboarding, boxing, football and gymnastics.
- The concept of "no car damage = no injury" is COMPLETELY false. Most cars can withstand collisions of up to 10 MPH and as pointed out above, only in collisions < 5 MPH are you less likely to be injured. Collisions that occur between 6-12 MPH cause the highest percentage of whiplash injuries (which is below the threshold of car damage in most cases). Also, the energy of the impact is transferred to the contents inside the car when there is no vehicular damage (that means you).
- Mild traumatic brain injury (MTBI) can occur in motor vehicle collisions even if the head does not hit an object inside the car, although it's more common when there is a head strike. The symptoms associated with MTBI are often referred to as "Post Concussive Syndrome."
- Approximately 10% of whiplash injured patients become totally disabled.

- Of the studies published since 1995, over 60% of whiplash patients required long-term medical care.
- Risk factors for long-term symptoms associated with WAD include: rear impacts, loss of the cervical lordosis curve, pre-existing degenerative arthritis, use of seat belts & shoulder harness (low speed impacts only), poor head restraint position or shape, non-awareness of the impending collision, female (especially long slender neck), head rotation at impact.

Whiplash Down the Road

Whiplash injuries of the neck and spine commonly occur in auto accidents. Even minor impacts with little vehicle damage can put significant stress on the spinal ligaments, disks, and delicate nerves. Some people get whiplash symptoms right after the accident (which is a very bad sign) but most people feel somewhat unscathed, at least initially.

It's important to think how spinal injuries can affect you over the long term. When ligaments are injured, there can be substantial changes over the years, such as arthritis and disk degeneration.

A study in the science journal SPINE (Dec. 15, 1994) looked at fifty patients with MRI and bending x-rays, one and five years after injury. The researchers found that neck pain persisted in 24/50 (48%) patients and radiating pain developed within 6 weeks in 19 patients or 38%. Radiating pain occurs when a disk protrudes and bulges onto a nerve root exiting your spinal column. In patients with these persistent symptoms, the MRI was helpful in showing the disk injury.

Although surgery is considered by many, most patients do well under conservative entail substantial risks, and how well it works is also subject to debate.

X-rays and palpation are used to see the posture of your neck and how the vertebrae move in stressed positions. These tests can help determine how your spine functions and whether the disk is injured and/or also if you have pre-existing signs of arthritis, which can impair how you resist and recover from trauma.

Chiropractic adjustments are directed at reducing pain and improving mobility in spinal areas that are blocked. In general it's important to keep your neck moving while you recover. Staying in bed and not moving the spine at all is not advised since this can impair recovery. Even patients with severe whiplash injuries can have some movements preserved and these should be encouraged.

Because symptoms and even disk disease can show up later, it is important to have a detailed neurological examination following a neck injury. Whiplash trauma is significant, especially when you consider how many patients still suffer years down the road with neck and arm pain. Getting diagnosed properly is the first step to determining what type of care will be best for you.

treatment after an auto accident in Lacey Olympia WA. It's important to consider non-surgical options first, since surgery does

Whiplash Injury and Cervicogenic Headache

Barbara is a 45-year old woman with two adult children. She is employed full-time as a sales clerk at the local mall. Her job is not physically demanding nor is it ergonomically challenging. Her job allows her to assume multiple physical positions throughout the day while she is assisting a variety of customers with a variety of needs. There is no required heavy lifting or prolonged postures.

Barbara is fit, with good muscle tone and posture. She stands 5 feet 4 inches tall and weight 120 pounds. Her exercise regime consists of walking several miles per day, nearly every day of the week, with a group of her friends.

Barbara has suffered with chronic headaches for 24 years. In addition, her headaches seemed to make her right shoulder ache.

Barbara's headaches began when she was involved in a motor vehicle collision that occurred at 21 years of age. She did not recall many of the details of the collision other than that she was the driver of a vehicle that was struck from the rear. The collision caught her by surprise and she remembers her head being thrown backwards. There was no loss of consciousness, and she did not experience being dazed, confusion, disorientation, or loss of any memory. The damage to her vehicle was minor, and she was able to drive away from the accident scene after exchanging insurance information with the man who was driving the striking vehicle.

Barbara did not experience pain or any other complaints at the accident scene. However, as the day progressed, she became aware of some minor neck stiffness. The next day was a different story. Barbara recalls that the next morning she was unable to pick her head up off her pillow without using her hands to assist her. Her neck was painful and stiff. And, she had a headache.

Barbara attributed her neck and head signs and symptoms to a "strain" injury caused by the vehicle collision she was involved in. She took some over-the-counter pain pills, and within a few days she was much improved.

However, about a week after the collision, Barbara became more aware that she still had a headache, and that it did not appear to be improving. Rather it seemed to be becoming more pronounced. The headache was located at the right upper posterior area of her neck and also around and behind her right eye.

Since being injured 24 years ago, Barbara has had to constantly deal with her headaches. They occur frequently and range in severity from annoying to debilitating. When she is suffering from a bad headache, she also notices an abnormal sensitivity to bright lights (photophobia). She notes that apparent triggers for her headaches range from certain neck movements to prolonged neck postures. Her headaches are always only on her right side.

Barbara's examination shows significantly reduced lateral flexion and rotation of the upper cervical spine on the right side. She is very sensitive to mild/moderate digital pressure applied to the suboccipital region and muscles. Importantly, her right-sided frontal (around her eye) headache can be triggered by sustained deeper pressure at the inferior margin of the right inferior oblique muscle. Recall, the inferior oblique muscle exists between the spinous process of the axis (C2) and the transverse process of the atlas (C1). (Two easily identifiable landmarks for a practicing chiropractor; see drawing page 10).

Barbara reports that she has consulted a number of medical doctors (general practitioners, not specialists) about these headaches, resulting in her taking a variety of over-the-counter and/or prescription medications. She reports that these drugs definitely help her, especially when her headache is severe. She states that she takes pain medicines for her headache 10-15 days per month. But, after developing some gastrointestinal bleeding from taking over-the-counter drugs, her primary care physician suggested she try the COX-2 inhibitor drug Celebrex. She has now been consuming Celebrex 10-15 days per month, reporting that it is quite helpful when she has a bad headache.

However, Barbara became concerned after hearing media reports of Celebrex and other pain medicines being associated with an increased risk of heart attacks. In addition, she reported that she was weary of having to consume pain medicines 10-15 days per month to function appropriately in her life. Barbara acknowledges that medicines she had been taking for her headaches were helpful, but that they had not cured her headaches, and her suffering had been going on for 24 years.

Barbara self-referred herself to our office as it was on her way home from work. She had seen no other chiropractors or physical therapists for her headaches. Our office was the first.

Whiplash Diagnosis

Whiplash is, by definition, the rapid acceleration followed by deceleration of the head causing the neck to "crack like a whip" forwards and backwards at a rate so fast that the muscles cannot react quickly enough to control the motion. As reported last month, if a collision occurs in an automobile and the head rests are too low and/or seat backs too reclined and the head moves beyond the allowable tissue boundaries, "whiplash" injury occurs.

When gathering information from the patient, this portion of the history is called "mechanism of injury" and it is VERY IMPORTANT, as it helps us piece together what happened at the time of impact. For example, was the head turned upon impact?

Was the impact anticipated? What were the weather conditions (visual, road conditions)? What was the direction of the strike (front, rear, side, angular, or combinations of several)? Did a roll over occur? Was a seat belt used (lap and chest) and were there any seat belt related injuries (to the low back/pelvis, breasts/chest, shoulder, neck)? Any head impact injuries with or without loss of consciousness (if so, how long)? Any short-term memory loss and residual communication challenges (post-concussive syndrome)? All of the answers to these questions are very important when determining the examination path, establishing the diagnoses, and determining the treatment plan.

We also discussed last month the WAD classification or, Whiplash Associated Disorders, which was coined in 1995 by the Quebec Task Force. Types I, II, and III are defined by the type of tissues injured and the history and examination findings. In 2001, the Quebec Task Force found that WAD II (loss of range of motion or ROM/negative neurological findings) and WAD III (both ROM loss and neurological loss) carried progressively greater risk of prolonged recovery compared to WAD I injuries (those with pain but no loss of motion or neurological findings).

Establishing a strong diagnosis allows for accuracy in prognosis and treatment plan recommendations. For example, in WAD II & III injuries, flexion/extension x-rays are needed to determine the extent of ligament damage as normally, the individual vertebrae should not translate or shift forwards or backwards by more than 3.5mm. Similarly, the angle created between each vertebra in flexion & extension should be within 11 degrees of the adjacent angles, and if that's exceeded, ligament damage is likely to have occurred. So often, ER records describe little to no information about the historical elements reviewed in the 1st paragraph and if x-rays were taken, they rarely include flexion/extension stress x-rays.

Headaches are another component of WAD. Here, the first three sets of nerves that exit the uppermost levels of the spine (C1, C2, and C3) innervate the head. When a patient describes headaches that start in the upper part of the neck and radiate up into the head, the distribution of the pain by history can tell us which nerve(s) are most affected. In the examination, applying manual pressure to the base of the skull can reproduce pain when a nerve is injured. Tracking these findings on a regular basis can tell us how the condition is healing. Chiropractic is at the forefront of diagnosis for WAD!

How Can I Get Hurt in a Low-Speed Crash?

Whiplash – or perhaps most accurately, "whiplash associated disorders" (WAD) – is a term that is applied to the MANY different types of injuries that can occur at the time of an automobile collision.

The cervical spine includes bony structures, ligaments (that hold bones tightly together), tendons (that attach muscles to bones), nerves (that allow us to feel and provides muscle strength), disks (that serve as shock absorbers between our vertebra), and other connective tissues that can be injured depending on MANY factors! The brain can also be injured (i.e., concussion) in a crash WITHOUT the head hitting anything! Individuals in car accidents can also experience seat belt-related injuries to the shoulder, chest, abdomen, mid-back, and/or low-back, as well as the extremities.

There are many factors that can increase your risk of injury including the size of the two vehicles (worse when a large vehicles strikes a smaller vehicle), the direction of the collision, the position of the head upon impact (worse if rotated), the size of the neck (females are at greater risk), the angle and springiness of the seat back, the position of the head rest (too low is common), and the amount of vehicular damage (or lack thereof).

The latter is the surprising part! You may have noticed when a racecar crashes, it's made to literally break apart until the only remaining piece is the cage that holds the driver. The reason for this is when a crash occurs, the energy of the impact (or "G-force") is absorbed by crushing metal or breaking away parts. If the vehicle is 'built like a tank' and no metal crushes or parts break off, the energy is transferred to the contents inside the vehicle – namely the driver and occupants!

Hence, the concept of "no vehicular damage means any injury" is actually quite the opposite! When low-speed collisions occur, there is no energy absorption by the crushing of metal or breaking away of parts. Hence, there's a greater chance of injury at low speeds when little-to-no damage occurs to the target vehicle!

Whiplash and Side Collisions

Whiplash is most commonly studied when it is a result of a rear collision where the occupant of the vehicle is injured from a flexion (forwards) and extension (backwards) whip-like mechanism of injury, but what happens when a T-bone type of impact occurs?

The answer to this question is quite similar to many of the factors associated with any collision: the size of the bullet vs. target vehicle, the speed at which the collision occurs, the deployment or lack thereof of the airbag(s), the position of the neck at the time of impact, the "build" of the patient (skinny/tall vs. muscular), the road conditions, the "springiness" and angle of the seat back, and so forth. Unique to side impacts is the location of the strike to the target vehicle (front, middle, rear) and perhaps more importantly, the lack of space between the occupant and the point of the strike as there is a relatively shallow "crumple zone" between the occupant and the side of the vehicle.

Probably one of the best examples of how side impacts from different angles can be appreciated is to think about what happens to a person when they ride the "Bumper Cars" at the local fair. Though many fairs have now banned that "ride," you may recall participating or watching those kids who were "having fun." When a bumper car is struck in a classic "T-Bone" manner in the front end, the target car is spun around and the occupant hangs on for dear life. Similarly, a side strike from to the rear of the bumper car spins the back end around. When the occupant is aware of the impending crash, they grip the wheel, tuck their head by shrugging their shoulders and make their body rigid and typically, do not get "whipped around" as much as those that don't anticipate the impact. Because the bumper cars don't dent or crush (that is, there is no plastic deformity where damage occurs, only elastic deformity where there is no damage or, no energy absorption by crushing of the car), ALL of the crash energy is transferred to the occupant or the contents. If a person has a purse lying on the floor of the bumper car, it can go flying out and spill all over. Similarly, the person who is unaware of the impending collision will "go flying," giving great satisfaction to the driver of the bullet bumper car.

When considering factors such as plastic vs. elastic deformity, side air bags, and the shallow crumple zone on the sides of motor vehicles, some manufactures stand out in their ability to protect the occupants in side impact collisions. Generally, those vehicles with a stiff side and roof structure have been found to be the best in protecting the occupant from injury by maintaining the survival space and dissipating the energy, or force, of the impact away from the occupant. Manufactures that stand out include Volvo, Mercedes, and Subaru. They have had the best design for decades and remain at the forefront for occupant protection in side impact collisions. The combination of energy absorbing side structure design and the side airbag has proven to be one of the most important factors in improving the crashworthiness in side impact collisions. Side air bags became popular in the 1990s. In 2012, more than 95% of all passenger cars sold in the US are equipped with side impact airbags as standard equipment.

Whiplash and PTSD

Whiplash injuries commonly result from motor vehicle collisions (MVC) and are caused by a sudden jolt that initiates a startle response that has been found to tighten the muscles deep inside the neck, which has been reported to increase the risk of injury to the joints and structures of the cervical spine. The amount of physical injury to the person is highly variable depending on many factors that include, but are not limited to, the size of the involved vehicles, speed at impact, amount of energy absorbed by crushing metal (especially the lack thereof), a slender female neck vs. shorter muscular male neck, the stiffness and angle of the seat back, the direction of the impact, head position (rotation is worse vs. straight), headrest position, and more. A cervical sprain/strain is commonly diagnosed in MVCs and these tend to resolve with chiropractic care, often without complications. However, this is not always the case. What factors are involved that result in one case improving and/or resolving but not another, especially when everything seems identical (or at least similar)? What does post-traumatic stress disorder (PTSD) have to do with MVCs? Is this a factor triggering a prolonged recover? Is PTSD commonly associated with whiplash injuries?

In a group of 112 PTSD whiplash patients, researchers examined the role of pain as well as pain-related psychological variables. Participants completed various questionnaires at three different time points after admission into a standardized multidisciplinary rehabilitation program. The findings revealed consistency with other studies showing injury severity indicators including high pain levels, reduced function / disability, and more severe scores on pain-related psychological variables in those suffering from PTSD following a whiplash injury. However, contrary to expectations, pain severity did NOT contribute to the persistence of PTSD. Rather, the most significant variables were self-reported disability, catastrophizing, and perceived injustice. These results suggest that early intervention that focuses on pain management and disability following whiplash might reduce the severity of PTSD but not the persistence of it. Rather, interventions that focus on resolving perceptions of injustice appear to be most important for helping patients recover from PTSD.

Similarly, another study looked at the factors that result in the best treatment outcome for patients involved in motor vehicle collisions (MVCs) with the subsequent onset of PTSD. Here, researchers carried out a review of prior studies to identify the risk factors associated with a prolonged recovery and a treatment strategy proposed to resolve the PTSD. They reported that at least 25% of study participants who sustained a physical injury developed PTSD and that the prevalence is most likely even higher in those who developed chronic whiplash.

Looking at what factors of PTSD are the most accurate predictors of duration and severity of PTSD, another study investigated the relationship between PTSD symptoms of avoidance, re-experience, and hyperarousal and their role in interfering with the resolution, the severity and duration of neck complaints following MVCs. Questionnaires were sent to 240 MVC injured patients that had initiated compensation claims with a Dutch insurance company and were evaluated three times – initially, at six months, and again at twelve months. They found that the hyperarousal symptoms of

PTSD initially had predictive validity for persistence and severity of post-whiplash syndrome at six and twelve months. They concluded that the hyperarousal symptoms of PTSD had the greatest detrimental effect on the severity and recovery of PTSD and focusing treatment at that was most important.

What Most People Don't Know About Car Accident Injuries

Whiplash (or WAD – whiplash associated disorders) can be defined by a sudden movement of the head and neck beyond its normal range of motion resulting in pain and stiffness and less often, numbness nd neck beyond its normal range of motion resulting in pain and stiffness and less often, numbness and tingling in the arms and hands. Prognosis is a term associated with a predicted outcome of a condition with the passage of time, either with or without treatment. A condition is considered "stable" when symptoms aren't changing and are not likely to change significantly over the next several months to a year. In general, recovery may depend on the severity of the injury. Usually, minor whiplash injuries will resolve completely within approximately one to two weeks, moderate whiplash injuries within approximately four to eight weeks, and severe whiplash may or may not completely "resolve." Rather, severe whiplash may result in a chronic condition which may lead to a permanent reduction or a complete loss of certain functions. There are "risk factors" that can result in either a prolonged recovery or just a partial recovery, regardless of the degree of injury which makes the process of prognosing whiplash cases challenging. Let's take a closer look!

There have been many published studies that have looked at the long-term prognosis of whiplash injuries using different approaches. For example, one study reported that reduced cervical range of motion was able to predict those less likely to fully recover after one year.

Another study broke down acute whiplash patients into seven risk levels using one-year work disability (total number of days missed from work) as the main outcome measure. The age of injured subjects ranged from 18-70 years and injuries varied between WAD 1 to 3 (WAD 1 = Pain but no loss of motion, primarily soreness; WAD 2: Loss of motion and muscle tightness/pain; WAD 3: Same as WAD 2 but WITH neurological problems like numbness &/or weakness in the arms due to nerve injury). The study evaluated a total of 483 women and 250 men within ten days of their motor vehicle collision (MVC). At the end of one year, a total of 605 participants completed the study and were given a "RISK SCORE" which included: a) initial neck pain/headache intensity; b) the number of non-painful complaints; and c) active cervical range of motion. When researchers compared the patients' RISK SCORE at the one-year mark to their work disability (number of sick days), they found a direct correlation between lower scores and lower work disability and higher scores and greater work disability. They concluded that this could be a valuable tool to assess a patient's ability to return to work following WAD injuries.

What Can I Do to Help Myself?

Whiplash or whiplash associated disorders (WAD) is a commonly used term for an acceleration-deceleration force applied to the neck often occurring in car crashes but may arise from a slip and fall, a diving accident, or other traumatic injury. The net result is an injury to muscles, ligaments, joints, and/or nerves in the cervical spine or neck region and possibly a concussion.

This month's article is intended to spotlight self-help strategies that YOU can do to help manage this afflicting condition. We HIGHLY recommend downloading "Whiplash Injury Recovery: A self-management guide" as it covers very important information in the 24 page PDF go to:

http://bit.ly/WHIPLASHGUIDE

It is authored by Professor Gwendolen Jull, the director of The Cervical Spine and Whiplash Research Unit, Division of Physiotherapy, at The University of Queensland. In her "message from the author," she writes the following:

"This booklet aims to assist persons who have had a whiplash injury on the road to recovery. It provides information about whiplash-associated disorders, an explanation of whiplash, and exercise program which has been proven to assist in reducing neck pain and advice on how to manage your neck to prevent unnecessary strain and to assist recovery. The booklet is a self-help resource to aid recovery and to supplement any care being provided by a health care practitioner."

In the table of contents, you will see whiplash defined, recovery information, and "helping yourself" topics followed by posture correction, proper sitting positions, lifting, carrying, and work instructions, as well as how to go about household activities. This 24-page guide concludes with exercise instructions followed by formal exercises, how often you should do them, and things to remember.

Here are some highlights:

1. Most people recover from a whiplash injury at different rates
2. Recovery ranges from days to months and occasionally one to two years – the majority recover fully
3. Research supports trying to continue with your normal daily activities – modify as needed and gradually return to normal work, recreation, and social activities
4. Be adaptive – make modifications to avoid flair-ups
5. Some activities hurt, but that doesn't automatically mean further injury. If you recover quickly, make modifications as necessary but continue the activity

6. You are your BEST resource in the recovery process (stay motivated to fully recover)
7. Stay active. Try to do as many of your normal activities as possible and gradually increase the intensity, frequency, and duration until normal function is returned
8. Try to keep working – work with your employer and co-workers so you can stay on the job
9. Don't skip simple pleasures – enjoy time with family and friends, participate in social outings, begin or rediscover a new hobby
10. Work with healthcare providers (like your doctor of chiropractic) to gradually introduce and increase exercises to regain motion, strengthen weak muscles, and improve function
11. Be aware of your posture
12. Modify activities to reduce strain during work and recreation
13. Be more active / less sedentary to PREVENT neck pain
14. Take breaks and change body positions throughout the workday
15. Arrange your workstation/desk (monitor position, keyboard /

mouse and chair "set-up") to be more ergonomic
16. Think about how you are sitting
17. Act as usual, be active, be aware (posture, taking breaks, etc.)
18. DO YOUR EXERCISES (modify according to comfort)
19. Follow the instructions during exercise training (avoid sharp/knife-like pain)
20. Communicate with your healthcare provider when questions arise!

The Whiplash Syndrome: Posture and Exercise

Whiplash can result from a number of causes, not just from motor vehicle accidents. A fall on the ice or a slippery floor, from a sports related injury, or even at the county fair on one of those rides that throws you around can result in the same type of injury. Whiplash occurs when the head is literally "whipped" either forwards and backwards or from side to side. It can include hitting the head but often does not. Symptoms vary considerably and therefore the term, "whiplash associated disorders" or WAD has been adopted, based on the clinical presentation of the patient and on the specific tissues injured. Common symptoms include neck pain, loss of motion, headache and sometimes arm pain or numbness resulting in difficulty driving, working, sleeping and concentrating.

Spinal manipulation of the neck has been found to be highly effective in the treatment of whiplash or WAD, and hence, Chiropractic is often the recommended first order of treatment for patients suffering from this condition. We have previously discussed the steps involved when presenting to a chiropractic clinic, from taking a detailed history and performing a thorough physical examination, and well as the many types of treatment options that exist. Exercise is one of the most important forms of treatment as they can and should be performed multiple times a day as directed by us, so that a return to normal function with no pain can occur as quickly as possible. Presented here are a few VERY EFFECTIVE exercises that we frequently give to patients suffering from WAD:

* For #3, ALWAYS apply a push or resistance with your hand through the FULL range of comfortable motion in that plane. That means, in one direction let the head "win" (like in arm wrestling) and when moving in the opposite direction, let the hand "win," (but don't let up pushing with the head). In other words, you are ALWAYS resisting against the movement in both directions moving as far as you can in both directions.

1	**Posture Correction**	A. Arch the back. B. Retract the shoulders and tuck in the chin. Hold for 10-30 sec. & repeat.		
2	**Chin Retractions**	A. Sit properly. B. Place your finger next to the chin. C. Retract head & hold 10 sec. & repeat.		
3	**Neck Strength Exercises**	A. Rotate RT using 10% Max. B. Repeat to LT hold 5 sec.		Repeat this moving the head Forwards, backwards, & sideways in a similar way!*

See What Our Patients Have To Say...

"Dr. David Warwick took the time to learn about my injury and recommend my options. I started with a back adjustment, and it just felt a little better immediately afterwards. I woke up the next morning and felt way better. I am now convinced I will continue my treatment until I feel completely healed. Glad I went here and met with Dr. Warwick."

"I came, hesitantly, to Dr. Warwick's office due to pain, numbness, and tingling down both arms and limited range of motion in my neck and shoulders. I was not familiar with chiropractic as a medical option, but was faced with an ongoing treatment regimen of shots in my neck and limiting my activities, possibly forever. I decided I was not ready for that and needed a more logical, natural way to return to health. Needless to say, there has been great improvement not only in my neck and shoulders, but also lower back – discomfort I had just gotten used to. Dr. Warwick's willingness to really listen and understand my interest in a natural solution to regaining my health and strength has been empowering. Dr. Warwick is a medical provider, teacher, and true healer. THANK YOU!!!

"After my auto accident I experienced frequent and mysterious headaches. But not so mysterious for Dr. Warwick. He was knowledgeable, kind, and thoughtful in explaining to me my situation. Since seeing him, my headaches are gone. I feel confident in the care Dr. Warwick skillfully provides."

"Dr. David Warwick took the time to learn about my injury and recommend my options. I started with a back adjustment, and it just felt a little better immediately afterwards. I woke up the next morning and felt way better. I am now convinced I will continue my treatment until I feel completely healed. Glad I went here and met with Dr. Warwick."

"WOW! I am pain-free for the first time in two weeks! Thanks so much to Dr. David Warwick for an amazing job. I have so far to go, but now I am on the right track. I have been telling people for years that proper setup of a guitar is crucial to it playing well, just as a front alignment and tune up is to a car. It will work without it, but no where near its potential. All this time, my spine has been a disaster. The first visit, I knew I was on the right track. Treated like a welcomed guest, not as a number, and walking away with less pain and increased mobility. I had forgotten it was possible! Thank you so much!"

"I went into to meet with Dr. Warwick today, having been worked on by several massage therapists and Chiropractors over the years. I had a long relationship with my chiropractor and was really just trying something new and networking (I am a massage therapist) BUT Oh MY! He adjusted me today, found things I didn't realize were going on, relieved pain I wasn't really fully aware of and changed my entire day by lifting my mood and making my stress tolerable. I ended up with a smile for several hours just because I felt AMAZING! I will be singing his praises from the mountain top, As for my other chiro, well thanks for the memories but I am now a client of Dr. Warwick! If he can do that on my first visit, I can't wait to see what regular visits will do!"

"I don't do these often, so those who know me also know how much weight this carries. Highlight of my day today was probably the most no-nonsense, hassle-free, and delightful visit to the offices of my friend Dr. David Warwick to get a checkup of my lower back pain. No lectures, no suggestions of 20 "preventive" visits, just an honest diagnosis, some great pointers, a quick and effective adjustment, and out the door I went. For anyone seeking a fantastic chiropractor, please give Dr. Warwick a call; more than a Doc, the man is a breath of fresh air!"

"Dr. David is a miracle worker!! I saw him after having no idea how I injured my back and had seen another chiropractor twice….. but within two visits Dr. David had me walking, sitting, and sleeping pain free. Thank you Dr. David…you are simply the best!!"

"I have been in pain for a very long time but I went Dr. Warwick, and he was the only one that has help me with my lower back pain. I will continue to keep on seeing him for as long as I can. Thank you, Dr. Warwick!"

"I have never felt better in years, I have suffered from neck pain for a long time. I have had numerous doctor visits and have always still had pain. I have been seeing Dr. Warwick and was pleasantly surprised of the relief I continue to have. I love, love, love the results!"

"I came in to see Dr. Warwick because I was suffering from Bells Palsy. Almost immediately I started seeing results. I have now been going to Dr. Warwick for 2 ½ months, and I'm 100% back. I contribute that completely to the chiropractic work I have been doing. Not only that but I found out my body was lopsided, and I feel so much better. I haven't felt this good in ten years!"

"Dr. Warwick is very kind, attentive and professional. He always asks how I am feeling and if the chiropractic work he offers is helpful to me and my health. I really appreciate his professionalism, care and knowledge. I would happily refer him to all my friends!"

"Dr. Warwick is so dedicated to your health and happiness. It has been a pleasure being treated by him and others on the staff.

I have suffered from back pain for several years. I have seen multiple chiropractors, doctors, massage therapists, and acupuncturists. I even had 3 back injections! All provided no relief. I saw Dr. Warwick ONE time and I was pain free for 12 hours, which was the first time I had been pain free in years! After 3 treatments I was pain free for a week! HIGHLY RECOMMEND!!

Today was my first time ever going into a chiropractic office, I was so nervous at first, but when Dr. David M Warwick talked to me about what was going to be done I was comfortable. He was very quick and gentle and the relief of 9 years of tension, misalignment, and stress in my neck, mid, and lower back was instantly gone. I would recommend him to anyone to go to. I seriously feel so much better for the first time in a long time thanks to him!

1st time ever to see a chiropractor & Dr. Warwick has done an amazing job with adjusting my lower back! He has been very explanatory & most of all patient with me as I learn the process for what needs to be done. I really like the option of either walking in or making an appt. online too!

Check Out Patient Reviews
Facebook: Warwick Chiropractic PLLC

REFERENCES:

The 2008 Decade Task Force (Spine, 2-15-08).

Crowe H. Injuries to the cervical spine. Western Orthop Assoc., San Francisco, CA, 1928.

Spitzer WO, Skovron ML, Salmi LR, et al. Scientific monograph of the Quebec Task Force on Whiplash-Associated Disorders: redefining whiplash and its management. Spine 1995;20:2S-73S.

Freeman MD. A review and methodologic critique of the literature refuting whiplash syndrome. Spine 1999;24:86-98.

Bogduk N. The anatomy and pathophysiology of whiplash. Clin Biomech 1986;1:92-101.

Kaneoka K, Ono K, Inami S, Hayashi K. Motion analysis of cervical vertebrae during whiplash loading. Spine 1999;24:763-770.

Panjabi MM, Cholewicki J, Nibu K, et al. Simulation of whiplash trauma using whole cervical spine specimens. Spine 1998;23:17-24.

McKinney LA, Dornan JO, Ryan M. The role of physiotherapy in the management of acute neck sprains following road-traffic accidents. Arch Emerg Med 1989;6:27-33.

Mealy K, Brennan H, Fenelon GC. Early mobilization of acute whiplash injuries. BMJ 1986;292:656-657.

Rosenfeld M, Gunnarsson R, Borenstein P. Early intervention in whiplash-associated disorders. A comparison of two treatment protocols. Spine 2000;25:1782-1787.
http://www.letamericaknow.com/view_feature_ms.php?orderid=110&issue=1 005

Public Health Impact: http://www.srisd.com/consumer_site/epidemiology.htm

C-Spine CMT for HNP: http://srisd.com/research.htm

Sitting biomechanics Part I & II: http://srisd.com/research.htm

Harrison DD, Harrison SO, Croft AC, Harrison DE, Troyanovich SJ: Sitting biomechanics, part I: review of the literature. JMPT 22(9):594-609, 1999.

Harrison DD, Harrison SO, Croft AC, Harrison DE, Troyanovich SJ: Sitting biomechanics, part II: optimal car driver's seat and optimal driver's spinal model. JMPT 23(1):37-47, 2000.

http://www.neuroskills.com/tbi/injury.shtml

http://www.emedicinehealth.com/whiplash/article_em.htm

http://www.medicinenet.com/whiplash/article.htm

http://wiki.answers.com/Q/What_is_the_Best_safety_feature_for_preventing_whiplash_in_a_car

http://www.mgasouthcarolinatesting.com/blog/?p=858

http://www.webmd.com/pain-management/news/20080122/whiplash-what-predicts-recovery

http://www.webmd.com/back-pain/news/20020520/hands-on-approach-best-for-neck-pain

http://brain.oxfordjournals.org/content/132/10/2850.abstract

http://www.aetna.com/cpb/medical/data/400_499/0453.html

Brain (2009) 132 (10): 2850-2870. doi: 10.1093/brain/awp181
First published online: July 16, 2009

http://kingstonchiro.net/custom_content/c_98785_whiplash_facts.html

http://www.spineuniverse.com/conditions/whiplash/facts-tips-about-whiplash

http://www.truckinfo.net/trucking/whiplash-statiscs.htm
    Dan Baldyga - Author
    dbpaw@comcast.net

    AUTO ACCIDENT PERSONAL INJURY INSURANCE CLAIM
    (How To Evaluate And Settle Your Loss)
    http://www.autoaccidentclaims.com

Harling L, Brison RJ, Ardern C, Pickett W. Prognostic Value of the Quebec Classification of Whiplash-Associated Disorders. Spine 2001;26:36-41;

NISSAN, M.; OVADIA, D.; DEKEL, S.; Whiplash Associated Disorders - Subjective Complaints vs Clinical and Objective Findings. A Retrospective Study of 866 Patients JOURNAL OF BACK AND MUSCULOSKELETAL REHABILITATION. 2002;16(1)39-43; Norris, S.H., Watt, I: The Prognosis of

Neck Injuries Resulting from Rear-End Vehicle Collisions. J. Bone & Joint Surgery. 1983;65B:608-611;

Hendriks EF, Scholten-Peeters GG, van der Vindt DA, Neeleman-van der Steen CW, et al. Prognostic factors for poor recovery in acute whiplash patients. Pain. 2005 Apr;114(3):408-16.

http://www.chiro.org/LINKS/FULL/Whiplash_A_Medical_Doctor_s_Review_of_the_Literature.html

http://www.webmd.com/a-to-z-guides/ringing-in-the-ears-tinnitus-topic-overview

http://www.docroberts.com/bg-274-tinnitus-and-chiropractic.aspx

http://www.ncbi.nlm.nih.gov/pubmed?term=tinnitus%20and%20chiropractic

http://www.injurytreatment.com.au/search-injury-information/neck

http://www.braininjury.com/injured.shtml
http://www.osteopathyspecialist.com.au/treatments/whiplash/

Emary PC.; J Chiropr Med. 2010 Mar;9(1):22-7.; PMID: 21629395; [PubMed] ; Free PMC Article

Vertigo, tinnitus, and hearing loss in the geriatric patient. Kessinger RC, Boneva DV. J Manipulative Physiol Ther. 2000 Jun;23(5):352-62. PMID: 10863256 [PubMed - indexed for MEDLINE]

Chiropractic treatment of temporomandibular disorders using the activator adjusting instrument and protocol. DeVocht JW, Schaeffer W, Lawrence DJ. Altern Ther Health Med. 2005 Nov-Dec;11(6):70-3. PMID: 16320863 [PubMed - indexed for MEDLINE] Related citations

Self-reported nonmusculoskeletal responses to chiropractic intervention: a multination survey. Leboeuf-Yde C, Pedersen EN, Bryner P, Cosman D, Hayek R, Meeker WC, Shaik J, Terrazas O, Tucker J, Walsh M. J Manipulative Physiol Ther. 2005 Jun;28(5):294-302; discussion 365-6. PMID: 15965403 [PubMed - indexed for MEDLINE] Related citations

Chiropractic care of a patient with temporomandibular disorder and atlas subluxation. Alcantara J, Plaugher G, Klemp DD, Salem C. J Manipulative Physiol Ther. 2002 Jan;25(1):63-70. PMID: 11898020 [PubMed - indexed for MEDLINE] Related citations

Case study: acceleration/deceleration injury with angular kyphosis. Kessinger RC, Boneva DV. J Manipulative Physiol Ther. 2000 May;23(4):279-87. PMID: 10820301 [PubMed - indexed for MEDLINE] Related citations
Manipulative Physiol Ther. 2000 May;23(4):279-87.

Colachis SC Jr, Strohm BR. Cervical traction: Relationship of traction time to varied tractive force with constant angle of pull. Archiv Phys Med Rehabil. 1965;46(12):815-819.

Deets D, Hands KL, Hopp SS. Cervical traction: A comparison of sitting and supine positions. Phys Therapy. 1977;57(3):255-261.

Ellenberg MR, Honet JC, Treanor WJ. Cervical radiculopathy. Archiv Phys Med Rehabil. 1994;75:342-352.

Frankel VH, Shore NA, Hoppenfeld S. Stress distribution in cervical traction: Prevention of temporomandibular joint pain syndrome: A case report. Clinic Orthoped. 1964;32:114-115.

Franks A. Temporomandibular joint dysfunction associated with cervical traction. Ann Phys Med. 1967;8:38-40.

Geiringer SR, Kincaid CB, Rechtien JR. Traction, manipulation, and massage. In: Rehabilitation Medicine: Principles and Practice. 2nd ed. JA DeLisa, ed. Philadelphia, PA: J.B. Lippincott Co.; 1993:440-444.

Glacier Cross, Inc. Patient Satisfaction Survey. Kalispell, MT: Glacier Cross; 1997.

Glacier Cross, Inc. What Healthcare Professionals Say About Pronex. Kalispell, MT: Glacier Cross; October 1995.

Harris PR. Cervical traction: Review of literature and treatment guidelines. Phys Ther. 1997;57(8):910-914.

Lawson A. Pronex Cervical Traction Device: Application and Effectiveness. Kalispell, MT: Glacier Cross; October 1995.

Olson VL. Case report: Chronic whiplash associated disorder treated with home cervical traction. J Back Musculoskel Rehab. 1997;9:181-190.

Saunders HD. Introduction: Efficacy of traction for back and neck pain. Phys Ther Perspect. 1997;117(5):53-54.

Sauders Group, Inc. Saunders Cervical Hometrac®: A Guide for Clinicians and Third Party Payers. Chaska, MN: The Saunders Group, Inc.; July 1998.

Shore N, Frankel V, Hoppenfeld S. Cervical traction and temporomandibular joint dysfunction. J Am Dent Assoc. 1964;68(1):4-6.

Van Der Heijden GJ, Beurskens AJ, Koes BW, et al. The efficacy of traction for back and neck pain: A systematic, blinded review of randomized clinical trial methods. Phys Ther. 1995;75(2):93-104.

Aker PD, Gross AR, Goldsmith CH, et al. Conservative management of mechanical neck pain: Systematic overview and meta-analysis. Br Med J. 1996;313:1291-1296.

Venditti PP, Rosner AL, Kettner N, et al. Cervical traction device study: A basic evaluation of home-use supine cervical traction devices. JNMS: J Neuromusc System. 1995;3(2):82-91.

Moeti P, Marchetti G. Clinical outcome from mechanical intermittent cervical traction for the treatment of cervical radiculopathy: A case series. J Orthop Sports Phys Ther. 2001;31(4):207-213.

Gross AR, Aker PD, Goldsmith CH, et al. Physical medicine modalities for mechanical neck disorders. Cochrane Database Syst Rev. 1998;(1):CD000961.

Boskovic K. Physical therapy of subjective symptoms of the cervical syndrome. Med Pregl. 1999;52(11-12):495-500.

Swezey RL, Swezey AM, Warner K. Efficacy of home cervical traction therapy. Am J Phys Med Rehabil. 1999;78(1):30-32.

McCarthy L. Safe handling of patients on cervical traction. Nurs Times. 1998;94(14):57-59.

Nakamura K, Kurokawa T, Hoshino Y, et al. Conservative treatment for cervical spondylotic myelopathy: Achievement and sustainability of a level of 'no disability'. J Spinal Disord. 1998;11(2):175-179.

Shterenshis MV. The history of modern spinal traction with particular reference to neural disorders. Spinal Cord. 1997;35(3):139-146.

Wong AM, Lee MY, Chang WH, et al. Clinical trial of a cervical traction modality with electromyographic biofeedback. Am J Phys Med Rehabil. 1997;76(1):19-25.

Saal JS, Saal JA, Yurth EF. Nonoperative management of herniated cervical intervertebral disc with radiculopathy. Spine. 1996;21(16):1877-1883.

Hoving JL, Gross AR, Gasner D, et al. A critical appraisal of review articles on the effectiveness of conservative treatment for neck pain. Spine. 2001;26(2):196-205.

Carlsson J, Jonsson T, Norlander S, et al. Evidence-based physiotherapy in patients with neck pain. SBU Report No. 101. Stockholm, Sweden: Swedish Council on Technology Assessment in Health Care (SBU); 1999.

Nachemson A, Carlsson C-A, Englund L, et al. Back and neck pain: An evidence-based review. Summary and Conclusions. SBU Report No. 145. Stockholm, Sweden: Swedish Council on Technology Assessment in Health Care (SBU); 2000.

Kjellman GV, Skargren EI, Oberg BE. A critical analysis of randomised clinical trials on neck pain and treatment efficacy: A review of the literature. Scand J Rehab Med. 1999;31(3):139-152.

Philadelphia Panel. Philadelphia Panel evidence-based clinical practice guidelines on selected rehabilitation interventions for neck pain. Physical Therapy. 2001;81(10):1701-1717.

Washington State Department of Labor and Industries, Office of the Medical Director. Pronex and Hometrac cervical traction. Technology Assessment. Olympia, WA: Washington State Department of Labor and Industries; August 5, 2002. Available at: http://www.lni.wa.gov/omd/TechAssessDocs.htm. Accessed August 7, 2003.

Verhagen AP, Scholten-Peeters GGM, van Wijngaarden S, et al. Conservative treatments for whiplash. Cochrane Database Syst Rev. 2007;(2):CD003338.

Bronfort G, Nilsson N, Haas M, et al. Non-invasive physical treatments for chronic/recurrent headache. Cochrane Database Syst Rev. 2004;(3):CD001878.

Graham N, Gross AR, Goldsmith C; the Cervical Overview Group. Mechanical traction for mechanical neck disorders: A systematic review. J Rehabil Med. 2006;38(3):145-152.

Vaughn HT, Having KM, Rogers JL. Radiographic analysis of intervertebral separation with a 0 degrees and 30 degrees rope angle using the Saunders cervical traction device. Spine. 2006;31(2):E39-E43.

Binder A. Neck pain. In: BMJ Clinical Evidence. London, UK: BMJ Publishing Group; May 2007.

Borenstein DG. Chronic neck pain: How to approach treatment. Curr Pain Headache Rep. 2007;11(6):436-439.

American College of Occupational and Environmental Medicine (ACOEM). Neck and upper back complaints. Elk Grove Village, IL: ACOEM; 2004.

Cleland JA, Whitman JM, Fritz JM, Palmer JA. Manual physical therapy, cervical traction, and strengthening exercises in patients with cervical radiculopathy: A case series. J Orthop Sports Phys Ther. 2005;35(12):802-811.

Graham N, Gross A, Goldsmith CH, et al. Mechanical traction for neck pain with or without radiculopathy. Cochrane Database Syst Rev. 2008;(3):CD006408.

Raney NH, Petersen EJ, Smith TA, et al. Development of a clinical prediction rule to identify patients with neck pain likely to benefit from cervical traction and exercise. Eur Spine J. 2009;18(3):382-391.

Haines T, Gross A, Burnie SJ, et al. Patient education for neck pain with or without radiculopathy. Cochrane Database Syst Rev. 2009;(1):CD005106.

Jellad A, Ben Salah Z, et al. The value of intermittent cervical traction in recent cervical radiculopathy. Ann Phys Rehabil Med. 2009;52(9):638-652.

Young IA, Michener LA, Cleland JA, et al. Manual therapy, exercise, and traction for patients with cervical radiculopathy: A randomized clinical trial. Phys Ther. 2009;89(7):632-642.

Van Zundert J, Huntoon M, Patijn J, et al. 4. Cervical radicular pain. Pain Pract. 2010;10(1):1-17.

http://www.google.com/custom?q=Whiplash+exercises&sa=Google&client=pub-7936790299585611&forid=1&channel=4703386245&ie=ISO-8859-1&oe=ISO-8859-1&safe=active&cof=GALT%3A%23008000%3BGL%3A1%3BDIV%3A%23336699%3BVLC%3A663399%3BAH%3Acenter%3BBGC%3AFFFFFF%3BLBGC%3AFFFFFF%3BALC%3A0000FF%3BLC%3A0000FF%3BT%3A000000%3BGFNT%3A0000FF%3BGIMP%3A0000FF%3BFORID%3A1&hl=en